THE COMPLETE
NUTRITION COUNTER

THE
COMPLETE
NUTRITION
COUNTER

LYNN SONBERG

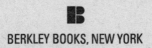

BERKLEY BOOKS, NEW YORK

THE BERKLEY PUBLISHING GROUP
Published by the Penguin Group
Penguin Group (USA) Inc.
375 Hudson Street, New York, New York 10014, USA

Penguin Group (Canada), 90 Eglinton Avenue East, Suite 700, Toronto, Ontario M4P 2Y3, Canada
(a division of Pearson Penguin Canada Inc.)
Penguin Books Ltd., 80 Strand, London WC2R 0RL, England
Penguin Group Ireland, 25 St. Stephen's Green, Dublin 2, Ireland (a division of Penguin Books Ltd.)
Penguin Group (Australia), 250 Camberwell Road, Camberwell, Victoria 3124, Australia
(a division of Pearson Australia Group Pty. Ltd.)
Penguin Books India Pvt. Ltd., 11 Community Centre, Panchsheel Park, New Delhi—110 017, India
Penguin Group (NZ), 67 Apollo Drive, Rosedale, North Shore 0632, New Zealand
(a division of Pearson New Zealand Ltd.)
Penguin Books (South Africa) (Pty.) Ltd., 24 Sturdee Avenue, Rosebank, Johannesburg 2196,
South Africa

Penguin Books Ltd., Registered Offices: 80 Strand, London WC2R 0RL, England

Every effort has been made to ensure that the information contained in this book is complete and accurate. However, neither the publisher nor the author is engaged in rendering professional advice or services to the individual reader. The ideas, procedures, and suggestions contained in this book are not intended as a substitute for consulting with your physician. All matters regarding your health require medical supervision. Neither the author nor the publisher shall be liable or responsible for any loss or damage allegedly arising from any information or suggestion in this book. The publisher does not have any control over and does not assume any responsibility for author or third-party websites or their content.

THE COMPLETE NUTRITION COUNTER

A Berkley Book / published by arrangement with the author

PRINTING HISTORY
First Berkley mass-market edition / August 1993
Revised and updated Berkley mass-market edition / January 2008

Copyright © 1993, 2008 by Lynn Sonberg
Book design by Laura K. Corless

A Lynn Sonberg book

ISBN: 978-0-425-21896-9

BERKLEY®
Berkley Books are published by The Berkley Publishing Group,
a division of Penguin Group (USA) Inc.,
375 Hudson Street, New York, New York 10014.
BERKLEY® is a registered trademark of Penguin Group (USA) Inc.
The "B" design is a trademark belonging to Penguin Group (USA) Inc.

PRINTED IN THE UNITED STATES OF AMERICA

10 9 8 7 6 5 4 3 2 1

ACKNOWLEDGMENTS

Special thanks are due to Deborah Mitchell for her invaluable help and advice in researching and writing this book.

CONTENTS

INTRODUCTION

Your search is over: This nutrition counter contains the most concise, up-to-date nutritional information on more than 4,500 foods you and your family enjoy. From artichokes to zucchini, apple pie to candied yams, this handy guide helps you target the foods that supply the nutrients that can lead to good health. It also allows you to discover which foods you may want to avoid, including foods high in bad fats (saturated and trans fats), cholesterol, calories, and sodium.

The foods are listed in alphabetical order and include both basic and brand-name items. If you are interested in bagels, for example, turn to B in the alphabetical listing and you will find information on fresh and frozen bagels. Similarly, if you want to learn about the nutritional content of foods served at fast-food restaurants, turn to FAST FOOD in the alphabetical listing, where the latest data from many of your favorite establishments are listed individually.

This convenient counter also makes it easy for you to compare similar foods. If you want to know how one brand of chocolate cookie compares with others, just turn to C for COOKIES and you can see the nutritional values for various name brands of chocolate cookies.

Convenience foods have become a very important part of today's society, so extensive information on frozen foods (including breakfasts, entrées, dinners, and sandwiches) is provided. To access these food items, just turn to FROZEN DINNERS & ENTRÉES. Here you will find information you need to choose healthful and nutritious meals you would prepare from scratch yourself at home if you had more time.

For each food item, the following information is provided: portion size, calories, protein (grams), total fat (grams), saturated fat (grams), trans fat (grams), cholesterol (milligrams), sodium (milligrams), calcium, iron, carbohydrates (grams), and fiber (grams). Calcium and iron are given as a percentage of U.S. RDAs (Recommended Daily Allowances), established by the Food and Nutrition Board of the National Academy of Sciences. These values are considered to be appropriate to meet the needs of most healthy Americans. They do not apply, however, to children younger than two years or to pregnant or nursing women whose nutritional needs are above average. Nutritional information on baby food is given in the percentage of U.S. RDAs for infants.

The bottom line is, if you want to maintain optimum

health and vitality while warding off everyday ailments and serious illness, you should know more about the food you serve yourself and your family. This nutrition counter is a convenient way for you to do just that.

Why You Need This Book

You know you should eat nutritious food and try to maintain a healthy weight so you can prevent illness and enjoy a sense of well-being and vitality, yet if you are like most Americans, you often fall short of those goals. Americans are heavier than they've ever been: An estimated 129.6 million Americans, or 64 percent, are either overweight or obese. A large percentage of Americans are also living with or are at serious risk for life-threatening diseases, including heart disease, stroke, diabetes, certain cancers, and high blood pressure—all diseases that are associated with diet. According to a study released in early 2004 by the Centers for Disease Control and Prevention, 400,000 deaths in 2000 were associated with poor diet and lack of physical activity. All this information points to one simple truth: If you improve your diet, you can improve your chances of preventing serious illnesses and, if you already have a medical condition, you can enhance your quality of life.

Although much information about nutrition is available from a wide range of media sources, it's not easy to find one comprehensive, convenient, easy-to-follow resource that provides the information you need to make healthy food choices. The Food and Drug Administration and the USDA have made nutrition labeling mandatory on processed foods, so you can read the labels on every item you buy at the supermarket when you shop. This is not always convenient, however; it takes time, sometimes the labels are difficult to read, and stopping to read labels in a crowded store may disrupt other customers as they shop. Labeling of fresh/raw fruits, vegetables, meats, poultry, and seafood remains voluntary, and often is not done.

The Complete Nutrition Counter makes label reading a snap—because it's all been done for you and information from those labels put into an easy-to-read alphabetical format. All the information is up-to-date on products available at this time. Nutritional information on fresh items, for which there are no labels, is also provided. You can use this book in the comfort of your home and write a shopping list based on items you read about in the counter. Or, you can bring the book along on your shopping trips. Either way it can help you discover how nutritious—or not so nutritious—your food choices are and help you make the shift to a healthier and more nutritious way of eating.

What Is a Healthy Diet?

Every five years, the U.S. Department of Health and Human Services (USDHHS) and the Department of Agriculture issue guidelines for a healthy diet. The

2005 Dietary Guidelines differ somewhat from previous guidelines in that they more vigorously emphasize the importance of reducing caloric intake, increasing physical activity, and making smart food choices from every food group. This new emphasis was instituted because two-thirds of Americans are either overweight or obese, and more than 50 percent get too little physical activity.

The new guidelines apply to Americans older than age two and recommend, based on a reference 2,000-calorie intake, consuming the following daily. Higher or lower nutrient amounts are recommended depending on your personal optimal calorie needs. (See Table of Serving/Equivalent Amounts on page xiv to help you choose serving sizes.)

- 4 servings of fruit
- 5 servings of vegetables
- 6 ounce-equivalents of grain foods, with at least half from whole-grain foods and the remainder from enriched or whole-grain foods
- 3 servings (cups) of fat-free or low-fat milk or equivalent dairy products (e.g., yogurt, cheese)
- 5½ ounces of meat, poultry, fish, or other protein equivalents (e.g., beans, eggs, nuts, seeds, tofu)

To help you gauge serving sizes based on the U.S. Dietary Guidelines, here is a list of serving sizes and their equivalents:

Table of Serving/Equivalent Amounts	
FOOD GROUP	**SERVING SIZE/EQUIVALENT**
Fruit	½ cup fresh, frozen, or canned fruit
	1 medium fruit
	¼ cup dried fruit
	½ cup fruit juice
Vegetables	½ cup cut-up raw or cooked vegetables
	1 cup leafy green vegetables, raw
	½ cup vegetable juice
Meat	1 oz cooked meat, fish, or poultry
	1 egg
	¼ cup cooked dry beans, legumes, or tofu
	1 Tbs peanut butter or other nut butters
	½ oz nuts or seeds
Dairy	1 cup low-fat or fat-free milk or yogurt
	1½ oz low-fat, reduced-fat, or fat-free natural cheese
Grains	1 slice bread
	1 cup dry cereal
	½ cup cooked rice, cereal, pasta

Some other recommendations from the USDHHS and USDA include the following. (The complete report can be accessed at http://www.health.gov/dietaryguidelines/dga 2005/document/):

- Total fat intake should be between 20 and 35 percent of calories, with the majority of fats from monounsaturated and polyunsaturated fatty acids, including fish, nuts, and vegetable oils
- Less than 10 percent of calories should come from saturated fat and trans fat
- Consume less than 300 mg per day of cholesterol
- Daily salt intake should not exceed 2,300 mg (about 1 teaspoon)
- For those who consume alcoholic beverages, they should do so in moderation—no more than one drink per day for women and no more than two drinks per day for men
- People who are overweight should work to achieve slow, steady weight loss by decreasing their caloric intake while maintaining an adequate intake of nutrients and increasing their level of physical activity
- To reduce the risk of chronic disease in adulthood, everyone should participate in at least 30 minutes of moderate-intensity physical activity on most days of the week
- To help manage body weight and prevent unhealthy body weight gain in adulthood, individuals should participate in approximately 60 minutes of moderate- to vigorous-intensity activity on most days of the week while not exceeding caloric intake requirements

Categories Covered in the Nutrition Counter

SERVING

Nutritional information on food labels is listed per serving, and this book follows suit by providing serving information as reported by the USDA and food manufacturers. Always check the serving sizes provided in this book and on the label. If you eat a larger serving, you will consume more calories and nutrients than those listed. This is a common error. You may, for example, typically eat three chocolate chip cookies and consider that to be one serving, yet the label may define a single serving as one cookie.

CALORIES

A calorie is a unit of food energy and represents the amount of energy needed to raise the temperature of a liter of water one degree centigrade at sea level. Everyone has his or her own caloric requirements necessary to maintain a healthy weight. This requirement is based on several factors, including activity level, age, and current health status. If you currently eat more calories than your body needs and burns, then you will likely gain weight. Generally, weight loss can be achieved if you decrease your caloric intake and/or increase your physical activity level. Tips on how to lose weight include:

- Using this book to help you keep track of your daily caloric intake and making sure you are getting adequate nutrients
- Increasing your intake of fruits, vegetables, and whole grains

- Limiting your intake of "bad" fats—saturated and trans fats—and instead focusing on "good" fats (see Total Fat later in this chapter)
- Increasing your level of physical activity (talk to your doctor before starting a new exercise program). If possible, exercise with a friend—it's more fun that way!
- Eliminating sugary foods and substituting fresh fruits for dessert

PROTEIN

Protein is one of the "big three" macronutrients (fat and carbohydrates are the other two) essential to maintain life and support growth. Proteins are composed of smaller components called amino acids, which are found in a variety of animal and plant foods. The meat and dairy food groups are the primary sources of protein, and the current serving size suggestions offer options for individuals who choose to avoid animal products when making protein choices. Vegetables and grains also contain a limited amount of protein. If you get your protein from nonanimal sources, it is recommended that you eat a variety of plant protein foods daily.

The World Health Organization recommends 0.45 grams of protein per kilogram (2.2 lbs) of ideal body weight per day, while the U.S. RDA recommends 0.8 grams as the maximum amount. Based on the recommendations of these two expert sources, if your ideal weight is 130 pounds, your minimum protein intake should be 27 grams and the maximum, 48 grams.

Most Americans consume too much protein from

animal sources. Because the body cannot store excess protein, it is eliminated in urine and feces. Before it leaves the body, however, it can cause stress on the kidney, which can be especially damaging in older people whose organs are less efficient. Because protein requires vitamin B6 to be metabolized and used by the body, excess levels of protein increase the body's requirement for the vitamin. When excess protein leaves the body, it may carry calcium with it, the loss of which increases the risk of developing osteoporosis.

TOTAL FAT

This category includes the total of the four main types of fats: saturated, polyunsaturated (which includes omega-3 and omega-6), monounsaturated, and trans fats. Fat is one of the "big three" macronutrients and is essential for life. However, "essential" does not mean you should consume great amounts of it. The Dietary Guidelines recommend Americans consume 20 to 35 percent of their calories from fat, although many experts argue that the 35 percent figure is much too high given the number of overweight and obese people in the United States.

Most Americans already eat more fat than they should, especially too much "bad" fat—saturated fat and trans fat. More about these two types of fats is explained below. The "good" fats—monounsaturated and the polyunsaturated fat called omega-3 fatty acid—typically are not listed on nutrition labels and so information about their values in foods is usually not readily available. You can deduce the amount of good fat in a food item by subtracting the sum of bad fats from the total fat value. The resulting number gives you a fairly accurate idea of the amount of good fat in the item, although the figure may also contain the polyunsaturated fat called omega-6, which is sometimes good, sometimes bad.

Although the various fats differ in several ways, they all provide 9 calories per gram, which is more than twice as much as the calories supplied by carbohydrates and protein (4 per gram). Thus fats can have a detrimental effect on your efforts to lose weight, improve overall health, or reduce your risk of heart disease and other medical conditions associated with high fat intake.

Despite the possibility of having a negative impact on your health, fats are also needed to maintain good health. Therefore, the best way to deal with fats in your diet is to balance them—eat fewer bad fats and switch to good fats. Here are some of the benefits of eating a balanced amount of good and bad fats:

- They help your body absorb fat-soluble vitamins (A, D, E, and K)
- They make you feel fuller, which helps you resist the temptation to eat snacks between meals and before bed
- They're good for your brain. Your brain is composed of 60 percent fat, and if you deprive your body of a sufficient amount of good dietary fats, you may experience emotional and mental effects, including poor concentration, faulty memory, and mood swings.
- Fats are necessary for optimal functioning of the immune system, which fights off infection,

promotes wound healing, and reduces the risk of cancer

- Skin, hair, and nails need dietary fat to stay healthy
- Fats are needed by the gastrointestinal system to help avoid constipation, bloating, and other digestive problems
- Fats help promote optimal nerve function

To help you balance your intake of good versus bad fats, you can include foods that are good sources of mono-unsaturated fats and omega-3 fatty acids, such as olive oil, avocados, salmon, herring, walnuts, and olives, and reduce your intake of bad fats (see "Saturated Fat" and "Trans Fat" below).

SATURATED FAT

This is the type of fat most often found in animal products, including meats, poultry, fish, and dairy products, as well as some tropical oils, such as palm and coconut. The liver uses saturated fats to manufacture cholesterol, which the body uses to produce hormones, among other uses.

A diet high in saturated fat is associated with elevated blood cholesterol levels, which can lead to heart disease and other serious medical conditions. This is why experts recommend that no more than 10 percent of calories be from saturated fat, and that people who are at high risk or who have heart disease limit their saturated fat intake even further. You can use this book to identify the amount of saturated fat in foods and to make healthier choices. At the same time, you can reduce the amount of saturated fat in your diet by eating more fruits, vegetables, and whole grains, choosing nonfat and low-fat dairy products, removing the skin from poultry, steaming and sautéing foods rather than frying them, and limiting your meat consumption to lean cuts while avoiding organ meats.

TRANS FAT

Trans fat is an artificial fat that is created when an unsaturated fat is bombarded with hydrogen atoms, resulting in a partially saturated fat. You can recognize trans fat on nutrition labels if you see the words "partially hydrogenated vegetable oil" or "hydrogenated oil," or "margarine."

Trans fat consumption is associated with significant health risks; there is evidence that it:

- doubles the risk of heart attack by increasing the levels of LDL (low-density lipoprotein) cholesterol (the "bad" cholesterol), decreasing the levels of HDL (high-density lipoprotein) cholesterol (the "good" cholesterol), and promoting the formation of blood clots, which increases the risk of heart attack and stroke
- increases triglyceride levels, which increases the risk of developing blood clots
- increases levels of C-reactive protein, a substance that causes blood vessels to become inflamed, resulting in an increased risk of heart disease
- damages cardiac metabolism, which can lead to heart disease
- harms the immune system, liver function, pregnancy and reproductive function, and insulin

response and function (especially a problem for diabetics)

- may increase the risk of developing cancer. Studies have found an increased risk of colon cancer associated with high consumption of trans fat, and a higher concentration of trans fat has been documented in the breasts of women who had breast cancer.

Trans fat, like saturated fat, is solid at room temperature and is made into margarine and shortening. These products are then used extensively in processed foods, including frozen foods, fast foods, fried foods, baked goods, snack foods, crackers, some margarines (usually hard stick varieties), and cookies.

CHOLESTEROL
Cholesterol is a waxy substance composed of fats and proteins. Although cholesterol is usually thought of as a completely "bad" substance, it plays several critical beneficial roles in the body, not least of which is that it is necessary for the production of many steroid hormones (e.g., estrogen, testosterone, progesterone, DHEA, pregnenolone, and vitamin D). Cholesterol comes from two sources: The liver manufacturers 3,000 to 4,000 mg of cholesterol per day, and you also get cholesterol from animal products. Similar to fat, cholesterol can be good or bad, depending on the type of molecule (lipoprotein) it attaches to as it travels through the bloodstream.

"Good" cholesterol is carried on high-density lipoproteins (HDL). HDL can help reduce serum cholesterol levels. Bad cholesterol is transported on low-density lipoproteins (LDL). Much of LDL cholesterol accumulates on the walls of the arteries, causing them to harden and become atherosclerotic, which can lead to stroke and heart attack. The Dietary Guidelines recommend that Americans limit daily cholesterol intake to less than 300 mg. If a blood test reveals that your cholesterol level is elevated (200 mg or greater), then you should limit your daily intake to less than 200 mg.

As you read through the counter, you will see that the foods with significant amounts of cholesterol are animal products such as meats, poultry, shellfish, eggs, and dairy products, as well as processed foods that contain these ingredients. You can reduce your intake of cholesterol by choosing low-fat dairy products and lean meats, limiting fried foods, and eating plenty of fruits, vegetables, and whole grains.

SODIUM

Table salt contains sodium and chloride, two essential nutrients in the diet. Most Americans, however, consume more sodium than they need. The 2005 U.S. Dietary Guidelines recommend that Americans consume no more than 2,300 mg (about 1 teaspoon, which contains 2,132 mg) of salt daily. This is slightly lower than the 2,400 mg recommended in previous years. It's important to limit salt consumption, as high intake has been linked to high blood pressure in some people—a significant risk factor for heart attack and stroke.

Even if you never lift a saltshaker, you consume sodium in your food, especially processed foods and fast foods, which can contain 50 percent or more of your daily recommended amount in just one serving! You can significantly reduce your intake of salt by using herbs, spices, and lemon instead of salt to season your food, not adding salt to pasta, rice, beans, or grains when cooking, checking nutrition labels for sodium content, removing the saltshaker from your table (out of sight, out of mind), and opting for more fresh foods rather than canned or processed, which are usually high in sodium.

CALCIUM

Calcium is a mineral that is critical for the development and maintenance of bone and teeth, and a host of other functions, including muscle contraction, immune system vitality, blood clotting, and cell membrane health. The main reason health experts stress the importance of sufficient calcium intake is for the prevention of osteoporosis, a brittle bone disease that most often strikes older women.

Calcium requirements change significantly throughout life, and in recent years the National Institutes of Health modified its recommendations to reflect those changes and the importance of getting enough calcium. For all adolescents and young adults ages 11 to 24 and for all pregnant or lactating women, the recommended daily intake is 1,200 to 1,500 mg. For women 25 to 49 and those 50 to 64 who are postmenopausal and taking estrogen, the requirement is 1,000 mg. Postmenopausal women 50 to 64 who are not taking estrogen, as well as women who are 65 years and older, should take 1,500 mg daily. Men ages 25 to 64 need 1,000 mg, while those 65 and older should get 1,500 mg.

Check the entries in this book to make sure you are getting enough calcium in your diet. Traditional sources of calcium include milk and other dairy products, but you may be surprised to learn that many vegetables, including broccoli, spinach, kale, and dandelion greens are excellent sources as well, along with salmon, sardines, and calcium-enriched foods such as orange juice and cereals. This book can help point you in the right direction when looking for foods that are good sources of calcium.

IRON

Iron is an important mineral essential to all cells in the body, as it carries oxygen through the body as part of hemoglobin in the blood and myoglobin in the muscles. Iron deficiency anemia is a common disease that occurs when there is not enough iron in the red blood cells. Pregnancy, blood loss (including heavy menstruation), and a diet low in iron are common causes of iron deficiency anemia.

Iron is found in a wide variety of foods and supplements, but the body's ability to absorb this mineral varies considerably. Iron is available in two forms: heme and non-heme. Heme iron is found only in meat, poultry, and fish and is absorbed more readily by the body than non-heme iron, which is found mainly in fruits, vegetables, nuts, grains, and dried beans. The ability of the body to absorb iron from non-heme foods can be increased if you eat foods rich in vitamin C (e.g., citrus, tomatoes, broccoli, strawberries) along with non-heme foods; if heme and non-heme foods are consumed together; and if non-heme foods are cooked in an iron pot. Consuming large amounts of coffee or tea with a meal, excessive consumption of high-fiber foods, and high intake of calcium along with iron can decrease non-heme iron absorption.

The Recommended Dietary Allowances for iron for non-vegetarian premenopausal women is 18 mg per day; for non-vegetarian men and postmenopausal women, it is 8 mg. Because vegetarian diets tend to be higher in fiber, the RDAs for iron for vegetarians are 33 mg for women and 14 mg for men. Consult this book to help you make sure you are getting enough iron in your diet.

CARBOHYDRATES

The main function of this macronutrient is to provide energy for the body, especially the nervous system and brain. Carbohydrates are broken down (metabolized) by the liver into glucose (blood sugar), which the body uses for energy.

At one time, experts divided carbohydrates into two groups: simple (including various uncomplicated sugars; e.g., white flour, white sugar) and complex (those composed of three or more sugars bound together; e.g., brown rice, whole grains, beans). They now know that carbohydrates are much more complicated than that. One measure of that complexity is something called the glycemic index, which measures how quickly and to what degree blood sugar levels rise after carbohydrates are consumed. Generally, however, simple carbohydrates cause blood sugar levels (and insulin levels) to rise sharply and rapidly (and have a high glycemic index) while complex carbohydrates result in a more moderate increase (and have a low to medium glycemic index).

It is more desirable to maintain steady blood glucose

levels, as fluctuating levels are associated with an increased risk of diabetes, heart disease, stroke, gallbladder disease, and some cancers. Fluctuating blood glucose levels also make it difficult to lose weight. One way the body responds to high glucose levels is to pump more insulin into the bloodstream. Rising insulin levels can also cause problems, as the insulin receptors in the cells become less sensitive to insulin over time, leading to insulin insensitivity, excessive production of insulin, and high risk of type 2 diabetes, heart disease, high blood pressure, stroke, and some cancers.

The recommended daily intake of carbohydrates is generally 50 to 60 percent of daily calories, although not all experts agree on these amounts. If you are interested in monitoring your carbohydrate intake, the values in this book can help you.

FIBER

Fiber is a noncaloric nutrient essential for promoting intestinal regularity, controlling blood glucose and cholesterol levels, and helping maintain weight and/or promoting weight loss. Fiber comes in two forms—soluble and insoluble—and most plant sources of fiber contain both types. The former is a sticky form found mainly in beans, dried peas, fruits, nuts, oats, and seeds. It binds to glucose in the intestinal tract and helps normalize blood glucose levels and also attaches itself to cholesterol, thus helping to reduce cholesterol blood levels. Insoluble fiber is coarse and helps promote regularity. It is found in many foods, including carrots, celery, barley, whole-grain cereals, and tomatoes.

The National Academy of Sciences has established that the adequate intake level for fiber is 38 grams for males 19 to 50 years of age and 25 grams for women of the same age. Currently, most adults consume about half of the recommended amount of fiber.

THE COMPLETE
NUTRITION COUNTER

KEY TO ABBREVIATIONS AND SYMBOLS USED IN THE COUNTER

c = cup
cont = container
f-f = fat-free
g = grams
med = medium
mix = mix only—not prepared
na = not available
oz = ounces
pc = piece
pkg = package
pkt = packet
prep = prepared
serv = serving
Tbs = tablespoon
tsp = teaspoon
< = less than
> = greater than

THE A-to-Z NUTRITION
COUNTER for BRAND-NAME
and WHOLE FOODS, INCLUDING:

- » CALORIES
- » PROTEIN
- » TOTAL FAT
- » SATURATED FAT
- » TRANS FAT
- » CHOLESTEROL
- » SODIUM
- » CALCIUM
- » IRON
- » CARBOHYDRATES
- » FIBER

FOOD NAME	Portion Size	Calories	
ACORN SQUASH, boiled, mashed	½ c	42	
ALMONDS			
Dry, roasted, no salt	1 oz	169	
Oil, roasted, no salt	1 oz	172	
ANCHOVIES, in oil, drained	1 oz	59	
APPLE JUICE			
Eden Foods, organic	8 oz	90	
Martinelli's	8 oz	140	
Minute Maid, frozen, prep	8 oz	110	
Mott's 100%, bottled	8 oz	120	
Mott's Plus Light Juice Beverage	8 oz	60	
Walnut Acres, organic	8 oz	110	
Apple white grape			
Minute Maid, frozen, prep	1 box	100	
APPLESAUCE			
Lucky Leaf Deluxe, cinnamon	½ c	100	
Mott's original	½ c	110	
Mott's unsweetened	½ c	50	
Musselman's	½ c	90	
APPLES			
Raw, with skin	med	72	
Raw, without skin	med	61	
Dried, sulfured	1 c	209	
APPLE BUTTER	1 Tbs	29	
APRICOTS, fresh	1	17	

Protein (g)	Total Fat (g)	Sat. Fat (g)	Trans Fat (g)	Chol. (mg)	Sodium (mg)	Calcium (%)	Iron (%)	Carbs (g)	Fiber (g)
1	0	0	0	0	3	3	4	11	3
6	15	1	0	0	0	8	7	5	3
6	16	1	0	0	0	8	6	5	3
8	3	1	0	24	1036	7	7	0	0
0	0	0	0	0	0	0	0	24	0
1	0	0	0	0	0	0	0	35	0
0	0	0	0	0	5	10	0	28	0
0	0	0	0	0	10	2	6	29	0
0	0	0	0	0	35	10	2	15	0
0	0	0	0	0	0	0	2	29	0
0	0	0	0	0	15	10	0	25	0
0	0	0	0	0	10	0	0	25	2
0	0	0	0	0	0	0	0	27	2
0	0	0	0	0	0	0	0	14	0
0	0	0	0	0	10	0	0	22	2
0	0	0	0	0	1	1	1	19	3
0	0	0	0	0	0	1	0	16	2
1	0	0	0	0	75	1	7	57	7
0	0	0	0	0	3	0	0	7	0
0	0	0	0	0	0	0	1	4	1

FOOD NAME	Portion Size	Calories	
Dried	1 oz	68	
Del Monte, canned, halves, drained	½ c	100	
Del Monte, canned, lite halves	½ c	60	
S&W, sun apricots	½ c	90	
S&W whole	½ c	120	
APRICOT NECTAR, organic (Santa Cruz)	8 oz	120	
ARTICHOKE			
Jerusalem, slices	1 c	114	
Birds Eye, hearts, frozen	12 pc	40	
ASIAN FOODS (canned, boxed); also see			
Frozen Dinners & Entrées			
Taste of Thai, Coconut Ginger			
Noodles, prep	1 c	280	
Taste of Thai, Red Curry Noodles, prep	1 c	280	
Taste of Thai, Pad Thai Noodles, prep	1 c	249	
Thai Pavilion, Authentic Pad Thai	⅓ pkg	230	
Thai Pavilion, Garlic Basil	⅓ pkg	220	
Thai Pavilion, Peanut Satay	⅓ pkg	210	
Thai Pavilion, Thai Green Curry	⅓ pkg	170	
ASPARAGUS, fresh, cooked, no salt	½ c	20	
Birds Eye, cuts	¾ c	20	
Birds Eye, spears	7	20	
Birds Eye, stir-fry, cooked	1 c	80	
Del Monte, canned, cuts & tips	½ c	20	
Del Monte, canned, spears	7	20	

Protein (g)	Total Fat (g)	Sat. Fat (g)	Trans Fat (g)	Chol. (mg)	Sodium (mg)	Calcium (%)	Iron (%)	Carbs (g)	Fiber (g)
1	0	0	0	0	3	2	4	18	2
0	0	0	0	0	10	0	2	26	1
0	0	0	0	0	10	0	2	16	1
1	0	0	0	0	25	0	4	22	1
<1	0	0	0	0	10	0	9	29	1
0	0	0	0	0	35	2	2	29	<1
3	0	0	0	0	6	2	28	26	2
2	1	0	0	0	55	4	2	7	5
5	7	7	0	0	680	2	4	53	1
4	8	4	0	5	820	4	4	51	2
5	2	.5	0	0	740	2	4	48	2
4	4	1	0	0	820	0	2	46	2
3	5	1	0	0	840	2	2	41	1
4	7	2	0	0	260	0	4	33	2
3	5	3.5	0	0	250	0	4	28	2
2	0	0	0	0	13	2	5	4	2
2	0	0	0	0	0	0	2	3	0
2	0	0	0	0	0	0	2	3	0
3	0	0	0	0	35	4	4	15	2
2	0	0	0	0	365	0	2	3	1
2	0	0	0	0	0	0	2	3	0

FOOD NAME	Portion Size	Calories	
Green Giant, cuts, no sauce, cooked	½ c	20	
Green Giant, canned spears	5	20	
Green Giant, canned spears, low sodium	½ c	20	
AVOCADO, California	1	289	
Florida	1	365	
BABY FOODS, Cereals			
Beech-Nut Naturals			
Barley	15 g	60	
Mixed	15 g	60	
Oatmeal	15 g	60	
Peaches Oatmeal & Bananas	4 oz	100	
Rice	15 g	60	
BABY FOODS, Dinners, juniors			
Beech-Nut stage 3			
Beef noodle	1 jar	97	
Turkey Rice	1 jar	95	
Gerber 3rd Foods			
Vegetables Chicken	1 jar	90	
Vegetables Ham	1 jar	102	
Vegetables Turkey	1 jar	90	
Heinz Junior-3			
Chicken noodle	1 jar	94	
Macaroni & cheese	1 jar	104	
Mixed vegetables	1 jar	56	
Spaghetti, tomato & meat	1 jar	116	

Protein (g)	Total Fat (g)	Sat. Fat (g)	Trans Fat (g)	Chol. (mg)	Sodium (mg)	Calcium (%)	Iron (%)	Carbs (g)	Fiber (g)
2	0	0	0	0	90	0	2	3	<1
2	0	0	0	0	430	0	2	3	1
2	0	0	0	0	210	0	2	3	1
3	27	4	0	0	14	2	6	15	12
7	31	6	0	0	6	3	3	24	17
1	<1	0	0	0	15	25	45	12	1
1	1	0	0	0	10	25	45	11	<1
1	1.5	0	0	0	15	25	45	11	1
2	1.5	0	0	0	13	0	35	18	2
1	0	0	0	0	10	25	45	12	0
4	3	1	0	14	29	1	4	13	2
4	2	0	0	7	136	4	4	16	2
3	2	1	0	12	129	5	3	15	2
3	3	1	0	5	148	2	2	15	2
3	3	1	0	7	151	3	3	13	2
4	2	1	0	15	133	4	4	15	2
4	3	2	0	10	129	9	3	14	1
2	0	0	0	0	15	3	3	13	0
4	2	1	0	9	128	3	5	19	2

FOOD NAME	Portion Size	Calories	
BABY FOODS, Dinners, strained			
Beech-Nut Stage 2			
Chicken Noodle	1 jar	75	
Sweet Potato & Chicken	1 jar	84	
Earth's Best, vegetables & turkey	1 jar	54	
Gerber 2nd Foods			
Beef Noodle	1 jar	71	
Broccoli chicken	1 jar	47	
Macaroni, tomato & beef	1 jar	69	
Turkey Rice	1 jar	59	
Heinz Step 2 Strained Foods			
Apples & Chicken	1 jar	73	
Vegetables & Bacon	1 jar	80	
Vegetables & Ham	1 jar	67	
BABY FOODS, Dinners, toddler			
Beech-Nut Table Time			
Beef Stew	1 jar	87	
Chicken, Noodle, Vegetables	1 jar	112	
Spaghetti, Tomato, Meat	1 jar	128	
Vegetable Turkey	1 jar	136	
BABY FOODS, Fruit			
Beech-Nut Stage 1			
Applesauce	2.5 oz	40	
Bananas	2.5 oz	70	
Peaches	2.5 oz	45	

Protein (g)	Total Fat (g)	Sat. Fat (g)	Trans Fat (g)	Chol. (mg)	Sodium (mg)	Calcium (%)	Iron (%)	Carbs (g)	Fiber (g)
3	2	1	0	18	26	3	4	10	2
3	2	1	0	12	25	3	3	12	1
3	1	0	0	5	23	3	2	9	2
3	3	1	0	9	17	1	3	9	1
4	2	0	0	7	21	5	4	4	3
3	2	1	0	8	43	2	3	11	1
3	1	0	0	6	23	2	2	9	1
2	2	0	0	6	14	2	2	12	2
2	3	1	0	5	55	2	2	10	2
2	2	1	0	6	18	2	3	9	2
9	2	1	0	22	587	2	7	9	2
6	3	1	0	48	316	2	4	15	1
9	2	0	0	0	609	4	9	18	0
8	6	0	0	0	568	8	6	14	0
0	0	0	0	0	0	0	0	9	1
<1	0	0	0	0	0	0	2	16	1
<1	0	0	0	0	0	0	0	9	1

FOOD NAME	Portion Size	Calories	
Pears	2.5 oz	50	
Beech-Nut Stage 2			
Applesauce	4 oz	60	
Bartlett Pears	4 oz	70	
Cinnamon Raisin Pears w/Apples	4 oz	130	
Mango Dessert	4 oz	90	
Mixed Fruit Yogurt	4 oz	100	
Peaches & Bananas	4 oz	70	
Prunes w/ Pears	4 oz	100	
Beech-Nut Stage 3			
Apples & Cherries	6 oz	90	
Applesauce	6 oz	90	
Chiquita Bananas & Berries	6 oz	170	
Fruit Dessert	6 oz	100	
Beech-Nut Table Time			
Apple Dices	4 oz	50	
Peach Dices	4 oz	50	
BABY FOOD, Juices			
Beech-Nut			
Apple Cherry (Naturals)	4 oz	60	
Apple (Naturals)	4 oz	60	
Guava Nectar (Stage 2)	4 oz	60	
Mango Nectar (Stage 2)	4 oz	70	
Mixed Fruit (Naturals)	4 oz	80	
BABY FOOD, Meat			

Protein (g)	Total Fat (g)	Sat. Fat (g)	Trans Fat (g)	Chol. (mg)	Sodium (mg)	Calcium (%)	Iron (%)	Carbs (g)	Fiber (g)
0	0	0	0	0	0	0	0	10	2
0	0	0	0	0	0	0	0	14	1
0	0	0	0	0	0	0	0	26	3
0	0	0	0	0	15	2	2	32	1
1	0	0	0	0	5	0	0	19	0
1	1	0	0	0	15	4	2	21	1
1	0	0	0	0	0	0	2	16	1
<1	0	0	0	0	0	2	2	26	2
0	0	0	0	0	0	2	2	20	2
0	0	0	0	0	0	0	0	20	2
2	<1	0	0	0	0	0	8	38	<1
0	0	0	0	0	0	2	2	24	2
0	0	0	0	0	0	2	0	13	1
<1	0	0	0	0	5	0	0	12	<1
0	0	0	0	0	10	0	2	15	0
0	0	0	0	0	10	0	2	15	0
0	0	0	0	0	0	2	0	15	0
5	0	0	0	0	5	2	0	15	0
0	0	0	0	0	20	0	2	20	0

Baby Food, Meat – Baby Food, Vegetables (Beech-Nut) FOOD NAME	Portion Size	Calories	
Beech-Nut Naturals			
Beef & Broth	2.5 oz	70	
Chicken & Broth	2.5 oz	50	
Lamb & Broth	2.5 oz	60	
Turkey & Broth	2.5 oz	90	
Veal & Broth	2.5 oz	50	
BABY FOOD, Snacks			
Beech-Nut, Arrowroot	3	30	
Beech-Nut, Banana Cookies	1	30	
Beech-Nut, Biter Biscuits	1	40	
Beech-Nut, Cheese Crackers	7	30	
BABY FOOD, Vegetables (Beech-Nut)			
Butternut Squash (Stage 1)	2.5 oz	30	
Butternut Squash (Stage 2)	4 oz	45	
Carrots & Peas (Stage 2)	4 oz	50	
Carrots & Peas (Stage 3)	6 oz	70	
Corn & Sweet Potatoes (Stage 2)	4 oz	90	
Country Garden Vegetables (Stage 2)	4 oz	50	
Green Beans, Corn & Rice (Stage 3)	6 oz	90	
Pasta Vegetable Medley (First Advantage)	4 oz	100	
Sweet Potato Soufflé (First Advantage)	4 oz	160	
Sweet Potato & Apples (Stage 2)	4 oz	70	
Tender Golden Sweet Potatoes (Stage 2)	4 oz	70	
Tender Sweet Carrots (Stage 1)	2.5 oz	30	
Tender Sweet Peas (Stage 1)	2.5 oz	40	

Protein (g)	Total Fat (g)	Sat. Fat (g)	Trans Fat (g)	Chol. (mg)	Sodium (mg)	Calcium (%)	Iron (%)	Carbs (g)	Fiber (g)
8	4	0	0	na	80	0	6	0	0
8	2.5	0	0	na	60	2	6	0	0
9	3	0	0	na	60	0	4	0	0
8	5	0	0	na	60	2	6	0	0
9	2	0	0	na	60	0	4	0	0
<1	1	0.5	0	0	35	10	10	5	0
<1	1.5	0.5	0	0	20	10	10	5	0
<1	1	0	0	0	10	10	10	8	0
<1	1	0.5	0	0	55	10	10	5	0
0	0	0	0	0	0	2	0	7	<1
<1	0	0	0	0	5	4	2	10	1
2	0	0	0	0	20	2	2	9	2
3	0	0	0	0	30	6	4	14	3
1	0	0	0	0	10	4	2	18	1
1	0	0	0	0	10	4	2	9	2
2	1	0	0	0	5	2	2	15	2
3	6	na	0	0	30	2	4	10	1
3	7	na	0	0	15	2	4	20	<1
0	0	0	0	0	5	2	2	16	1
0	0	0	0	0	10	2	2	17	1
0	0	0	0	0	20	2	0	6	1
1	0	0	0	0	0	2	2	7	2

FOOD NAME	Portion Size	Calories
Tender Sweet Peas (Stage 2)	4 oz	70
Tender Young Green Beans (Stage 2)	4 oz	45
BACON		
Hormel, Canadian	2 oz	68
Oscar Mayer, center cut	½ oz	50
Oscar Mayer, hearty thick cut	¾ oz	60
Oscar Mayer, ready to serve	½ oz	70
Oscar Mayer, ready to serve, Canadian	1¾ oz	60
Oscar Mayer, traditional	½ oz	70
BACON SUBSTITUTE		
Morningstar Farms, strips	2 strips	60
Yves, Canadian Veggie Bacon	4 g	80
BAGELS		
Lender's, blueberry	One 4"	264
Pepperidge Farm, cinnamon-raisin	1	270
Pepperidge Farm, plain	1	260
Pepperidge Farm, whole wheat	1	250
Sara Lee		
Apple Cinnamon	1 4-oz	310
Banana Walnut	1 4-oz	350
Blueberry Jr.	1	70
Blueberry, toaster size	1	160
Cinnamon Raisin, toaster size	1	160
Cranberry Orange	1 4-oz	310
Heart Healthy, 100% whole wheat	1	220

Protein (g)	Total Fat (g)	Sat. Fat (g)	Trans Fat (g)	Chol. (mg)	Sodium (mg)	Calcium (%)	Iron (%)	Carbs (g)	Fiber (g)
2	0	0	0	0	5	4	6	12	3
1	0	0	0	0	0	6	6	8	2
9	3	1	0	27	569	0	3	1	0
4	4	2	0	15	270	-	-	0	0
4	5	1.5	0	10	250	0	0	0	0
5	5	2	0	15	220	-	-	0	0
9	2	1	0	30	480	0	0	1	0
4	6	2	0	15	290	0	0	0	0
2	4.5	0.5	0	0	220	0	0	2	0
17	0	0.5	0	0	480	2	25	1	0
11	2	0	0	0	427	6	10	53	2
8	1	0	0	0	450	15	15	57	3
9	1	0	0	0	500	8	15	54	3
11	1.5	0	0	0	450	15	15	49	6
11	1.5	0	0	0	430	15	15	64	3
12	7	2	0	0	440	14	10	61	4
3	0	0	0	0	140	2	2	15	<1
6	0.5	0	0	0	310	6	8	34	1
6	0.5	0	0	0	300	6	8	33	1
11	1.5	0	0	0	430	14	14	64	3
11	1.5	0	0	0	480	10	15	47	6

FOOD NAME	Portion Size	Calories	
Honey Wheat, toaster size	1	250	
Onion, deluxe	1	260	
Onion, toaster size	1	160	
Plain, toaster size	1	160	
Sun-Dried Tomato & Basil	1	300	
BANANA, raw	One 7"	105	
Banana Chips	1 oz	147	
BARBEQUE SAUCE			
Heinz Jack Daniels Tennessee	2 Tbs	45	
Heinz Jack Daniels, steak sauce	1 oz	19	
Hunt's, Original, Bold	2 Tbs	60	
Hunt's, Honey Hickory	2 Tbs	60	
Kraft, Hickory Smoke	2 Tbs	40	
Kraft, Original	2 Tbs	40	
Kraft, Thick Spicy Brown Sugar	2 Tbs	60	
BARLEY, cooked	1 c	193	
BASS, cooked, dry heat	3 oz	105	
BEANS, baked			
B&M, Maple Flavor	½ c	145	
Bush's, Boston Recipe	½ c	150	
Campbell's, Pork and Beans	½ c	140	
Campbell's, Brown Sugar & Bacon	½ c	160	
S&W, Country BBQ	½ c	140	
S&W, Honey Mustard	½ c	140	
S&W, Sweet Bacon	½ c	140	

Protein (g)	Total Fat (g)	Sat. Fat (g)	Trans Fat (g)	Chol. (mg)	Sodium (mg)	Calcium (%)	Iron (%)	Carbs (g)	Fiber (g)
9	1	0	0	0	397	20	15	50	4
8	1	0	0	0	470	10	10	51	2
6	1	0	0	0	300	6	6	33	1
6	0.5	0	0	0	320	6	8	33	1
11	1.5	0	0	0	480	10	15	61	2
1	0	0	0	0	1	1	2	27	3
1	9	8	0	0	2	1	2	16	2
0	0	0	0	0	420	0	0	9	0
0	0	0	0	0	360	0	0	4	0
0	0	0	0	0	280	0	0	15	<1
0	0	0	0	0	280	0	0	15	<1
0	0	0	0	0	420	0	0	9	0
0	0	0	0	0	420	0	0	11	0
0	0	0	0	0	350	0	0	15	0
4	0	0	0	0	5	2	12	44	6
19	3	1	0	88	75	2	5	0	0
6	1	0	0	0	340	8	15	28	6
6	1	0	0	0	440	8	25	31	5
6	1.5	0.5	0	<5	440	4	8	25	7
5	2.5	0.5	0	<5	470	4	8	30	8
6	0.5	0	0	0	510	6	10	28	6
6	0.5	0	0	0	660	8	10	28	6
5	0.5	0	0	0	510	6	10	29	6

FOOD NAME	Portion Size	Calories	
Van Camp's, Bacon & Brown Sugar	½ c	140	
BEANS, other			
Adzuki, fresh, cooked w/salt	1 c	294	
Black, fresh, cooked w/salt	1 c	227	
Great Northern, cooked w/salt	1 c	209	
Navy, cooked w/salt	1 c	255	
Eden Organic, Adzuki	½ c	110	
Eden Organic, black	½ c	110	
Eden Organic, kidney	½ c	100	
Eden Organic, navy	½ c	110	
Eden Organic, pinto	½ c	110	
Eden Organic, soybean (black)	½ c	120	
S&W, black	½ c	70	
S&W, kidney	½ c	100	
S&W, white	½ c	80	
BEEF			
Bottom sirloin, lean & fat, roasted	3 oz	177	
Bottom sirloin, lean, selected, roasted	3 oz	153	
Brisket, lean & fat, choice, braised, flat half	3 oz	186	
Brisket, lean, choice, braised, flat half	3 oz	180	
Chuck arm pot roast, lean & fat, braised, choice	3 oz	264	
Chuck arm pot roast, lean, braised, choice	3 oz	180	
Chuck blade roast, lean & fat, choice, braised	3 oz	296	
Chuck blade roast, lean, choice, braised	3 oz	225	

Protein (g)	Total Fat (g)	Sat. Fat (g)	Trans Fat (g)	Chol. (mg)	Sodium (mg)	Calcium (%)	Iron (%)	Carbs (g)	Fiber (g)
7	1	0	0	0	540	6	na	30	6
17	0	0	0	0	561	6	26	57	17
15	0	0	0	0	408	5	20	41	15
15	0	0	0	0	421	12	21	37	12
15	1	0	0	0	431	13	24	47	19
7	0	0	0	0	10	4	10	19	5
7	1	0	0	0	15	6	10	18	6
8	0	0	0	0	15	0	8	18	10
7	0	0	0	0	15	8	10	20	7
8	1	0	0	0	15	6	10	18	6
11	6	1	0	0	30	8	15	8	7
5	0	0	0	0	480	6	10	17	6
7	0.5	0	0	0	460	8	10	23	6
7	0.5	0	0	0	440	6	8	19	6
21	9	3	0	72	45	3	9	0	0
24	6	3	0	51	48	3	9	0	0
27	9	3	0	39	45	0	12	0	0
27	6	3	0	69	45	0	12	0	0
24	18	6	0	87	39	0	12	0	0
28	7	2	0	65	46	1	14	0	0
23	22	9	0	88	55	1	15	0	0
26	12	5	0	90	60	1	17	0	0

FOOD NAME	Portion Size	Calories	
Chuck shoulder, lean & fat, choice, grilled	3 oz	156	
Chuck shoulder, lean, choice, grilled	3 oz	155	
Corned beef brisket, cooked	3 oz	213	
Filet mignon, lean & fat, broiled	3 oz	270	
Filet mignon, lean, broiled	3 oz	197	
Ground, 70% lean, patty pan broiled	3 oz	202	
Ground, 85% lean, patty, baked	3 oz	204	
Ground, 95% lean, patty, baked	3 oz	148	
Liver, panfried	3 oz	142	
London broil, lean & fat, choice, grilled	3 oz	162	
Prime rib, lean & fat, choice, roasted	3 oz	305	
Rib eye, lean & fat, select, broiled	3 oz	195	
Rib eye, lean, select, broiled	3 oz	153	
Round, bottom, lean & fat, choice, roasted	3 oz	168	
Round, bottom, lean, choice, roasted	3 oz	157	
Short loin, porterhouse, lean & fat, choice, broiled	3 oz	241	
Short loin, porterhouse, lean, choice, broiled	3 oz	190	
Top sirloin, lean & fat, choice, broiled	3 oz	186	
Top sirloin, lean, choice, broiled	3 oz	160	
BEEF SUBSTITUTES			
Amy's Kitchen, All American burger	1	120	
Amy's Kitchen, California veggie burger	1	140	
Amy's Kitchen, Chicago veggie burger	1	160	
Amy's Kitchen, Texas veggie burger	1	120	

Protein (g)	Total Fat (g)	Sat. Fat (g)	Trans Fat (g)	Chol. (mg)	Sodium (mg)	Calcium (%)	Iron (%)	Carbs (g)	Fiber (g)
22	7	3	0	63	50	0	12	0	0
22	7	2	0	65	51	0	13	0	0
15	16	5	0	83	964	1	9	0	0
21	20	8	0	73	50	1	15	0	0
24	11	4	0	71	54	1	17	0	0
19	13	5	1	66	78	3	11	0	0
22	12	5	1	77	54	2	13	0	0
23	5	2	0	62	49	1	14	0	0
21	4	1	0	309	62	0	28	4	0
23	7	3	0	66	48	0	14	0	0
19	25	10	0	71	54	1	11	0	0
24	12	3	0	81	51	3	9	0	0
24	6	3	0	51	54	3	9	0	0
24	9	3	0	90	30	0	9	0	0
23	6	2	0	88	31	1	11	0	0
20	17	6	0	59	55	1	14	0	0
22	11	4	0	55	59	1	15	0	0
24	9	3	0	66	48	3	9	0	0
26	6	2	0	56	54	1	10	0	0
10	3	0	0	0	390	4	10	15	3
6	5	0.5	0	0	430	2	8	19	4
10	5	1.5	0	5	390	8	20	14	3
12	2.5	0	0	0	350	4	10	14	3

Beef Substitutes FOOD NAME	Portion Size	Calories	
Boca Burgers			
Grilled, All American	1	90	
Grilled, Vegetable Burger	1	70	
Organic Cheeseburger	1	120	
Organic Garden Vegetable	1	130	
Organic Original	1	100	
Organic Roasted Garlic	1	130	
Organic Vegan	1	100	
Roasted Garlic	1	130	
Roasted Onion	1	130	
Morningstar Farms			
Grillers, Vegan	1	100	
Grillers, Prime Veggie	1	170	
Garden Veggie	1	100	
Mushroom Lover's Burger	1	110	
Spicy Black Bean	1	140	
Steak Strips	12 strips	140	
Worthington (canned)			
Redi-Burger patties	5/8"	120	
Tender Rounds	6 pc	120	
Vege-Burger	¼ c	60	
Vegetarian Burger	¼ c	70	
Worthington (frozen)			
Dinner Roast	¾" slice	180	
Meatless Corned Beef	3 slices	140	

Protein (g)	Total Fat (g)	Sat. Fat (g)	Trans Fat (g)	Chol. (mg)	Sodium (mg)	Calcium (%)	Iron (%)	Carbs (g)	Fiber (g)
14	3	1	0	5	280	15	10	4	3
12	1	0	0	5	300	6	10	6	4
15	4.5	2	0	5	650	0	8	7	5
15	3	0	0	0	400	10	10	9	4
18	1	0	0	0	390	8	40	8	5
16	3	0.5	0	0	470	10	8	9	4
13	2.5	0	0	0	470	10	8	9	4
16	3	0.5	0	0	470	10	8	9	4
15	3	0	0	0	420	15	10	10	4
12	2.5	0	0	0	280	4	10	7	4
17	9	1	0	0	360	2	8	4	2
10	2.5	0.5	0	0	350	4	4	9	4
7	6	1	0	0	220	0	4	8	<1
12	4	0.5	0	0	320	4	10	15	3
23	3	0.5	0	0	720	4	30	5	1
18	2.5	0.5	0	0	450	0	6	7	4
13	4.5	0.5	0	0	340	2	6	6	1
12	0.5	0	0	0	130	0	2	2	2
10	1.5	0	0	0	250	0	8	3	1
14	11	1.5	0	0	580	2	10	6	3
10	9	1	0	0	460	0	10	5	0

Beef Substitutes – Biscuits, refrigerated (Pillsbury) FOOD NAME	Portion Size	Calories	
Meatless Smoked Beef	3 slices	130	
Swiss Stake	1 pc	130	
Yves			
Good Veggie Burger	1	111	
Prime Veggie Burger	1	120	
Veggie Bistro Burger	1	140	
Veggie Ground Round, Mexican	2 oz	85	
Veggie Ground Round, Original	2 oz	58	
Veggie "Neatballs"	60 g	74	
BEER, regular	12 oz	153	
Lite	12 oz	103	
BEETS, fresh, boiled, sliced	½ c	37	
Del Monte, canned, sliced	½ c	35	
Del Monte, pickled	½ c	80	
BISCUITS, box/mix (Bisquick)			
Complete Buttermilk, mix	⅓ c	150	
Complete Cheese Garlic, mix	⅓ c	160	
Heart Smart, mix	⅓ c	140	
Honey Butter, mix	⅓ c	160	
Original, mix	⅓ c	160	
BISCUITS, refrigerated (Pillsbury)			
Country Style	3	150	
Freezer to Oven, Buttermilk	1	180	
Freezer to Oven, Cheddar Garlic	1	190	
Freezer to Oven, Southern	1	180	

Protein (g)	Total Fat (g)	Sat. Fat (g)	Trans Fat (g)	Chol. (mg)	Sodium (mg)	Calcium (%)	Iron (%)	Carbs (g)	Fiber (g)
11	7	1	0	0	510	2	10	7	<1
9	6	1	0	0	430	0	4	9	3
12	4	0	0	0	470	na	29	7	3
11	4	0	0	0	450	6	25	9	3
13	5	0	0	0	530	8	20	11	3
11	2.5	0	0	0	303	na	20	5	3
10	0	0	0	0	267	na	18	4	na
13	2	0	0	0	336	na	23	5	2
2	0	0	0	0	14	1	0	13	0
1	0	0	0	0	0	1	1	6	0
1	0	0	0	0	65	1	4	8	2
1	0	0	0	0	290	0	2	8	2
1	0	0	0	0	380	0	2	19	2
2	7	2.5	1.5	0	370	4	6	21	<1
2	7	2.5	2.5	0	350	4	6	22	<1
3	2.5	0	0	0	430	15	8	27	<1
2	2.5	2	2	0	320	2	4	23	<1
3	6	1.5	1.5	0	490	4	6	26	na
4	2	0	0	0	570	0	8	29	1
4	9	2.5	4	0	560	2	6	21	<1
4	10	3.5	4	10	700	6	6	20	<1
4	9	2.5	4	0	560	2	6	21	<1

Biscuits, refrigerated (Pillsbury) – Bouillon/Broth FOOD NAME	Portion Size	Calories	
Grands, Butter Tastin'	1	190	
Grands, Crescent	1	270	
Grands, Extra Rich	1	210	
Grands, Flaky Layers, Buttermilk	1	190	
Golden Layers, Flaky	1	110	
Microwave Butter Tastin'	1	200	
BLACKBERRIES, fresh	1 c	62	
BLUEBERRIES, fresh	1 c	83	
Cascadian Farm, frozen	1 c	70	
Dole, frozen	1 c	70	
Dole, frozen, wild	1 c	70	
BLUEFISH, baked	3 oz	135	
BOK CHOY, cooked, shredded	1 c	20	
BOLOGNA			
Louis Rich, turkey bologna	1 slice	52	
Oscar Mayer, beef	1 slice	88	
Oscar Mayer, beef light	1 slice	56	
Oscar Mayer, fat-free	1 slice	20	
BOUILLON/BROTH			
College Inn			
Beef	1 c	25	
Beef, French Onion Style	1 c	15	
Chicken, 99% f-f	1 c	15	
Chicken w/Lemon & Herb	1 c	15	
Garden Vegetable	1 c	25	

Protein (g)	Total Fat (g)	Sat. Fat (g)	Trans Fat (g)	Chol. (mg)	Sodium (mg)	Calcium (%)	Iron (%)	Carbs (g)	Fiber (g)
4	9	3	3	0	590	4	8	24	<1
5	15	3	5	0	510	2	8	29	<1
4	10	3.5	4	0	580	4	8	26	<1
4	9	2	3.5	0	550	2	6	24	<1
2	4.5	1	1.5	0	360	0	4	14	0
4	10	2.5	4	0	630	2	6	14	0
2	1	0	0	0	1	4	5	14	8
1	0	0	0	0	1	1	2	21	3
1	1	0	0	0	0	0	2	17	4
0	1	0	0	0	0	0	0	17	4
0	0	0	0	0	15	6	0	16	6
22	5	1	0	65	65	1	3	0	0
3	0	0	0	0	58	16	10	3	2
3	4	1	0	19	302	3	3	1	0
3	8	4	0	18	330	0	2	1	0
3	4	2	0	12	322	0	2	2	0
3	0	0	0	10	250	2	0	2	0
<1	1	0	0	0	900	2	20	0	0
4	0	0	0	0	850	0	0	0	0
1	1	0	0	0	930	0	0	0	0
1	1	0	0	0	715	0	0	0	0
0	0	0	0	0	590	0	0	6	0

FOOD NAME	Portion Size	Calories	
Turkey	1 c	20	
HerbOx, Chicken, regular	1 cube	5	
HerbOx, Chicken, sodium-free	1 cube	10	
Imagine			
Organic Beef Broth	8 oz	20	
Organic Free-Range Chicken	8 oz	10	
Organic Low-Sodium Vegetable Broth	8 oz	20	
Organic No Chicken Broth	8 oz	10	
Organic Vegetable Broth	8 oz	20	
Tyson Beef	1 cube	4	
Tyson Chicken	1 cube	4	
BRAZIL NUTS, unblanched, dried	1 oz	185	
BREAD			
Arnold			
Carb Country 100% Whole Wheat	1 slice	60	
Stone Ground 100% Whole Wheat	1 slice	70	
Stone Ground, Multigrain	1 slice	70	
Whole Grain Classics, 12-grain	1 slice	110	
Whole Grain Classics, 100% Whole Wheat	1 slice	90	
Country Classics, Oatnut	1 slice	110	
Country Classics, Oat Bran	1 slice	100	
Raisin Cinnamon	1 slice	100	
Real Jewish Rye	1 slice	90	
Earth Grains			
Buttermilk	1 slice	110	

Protein (g)	Total Fat (g)	Sat. Fat (g)	Trans Fat (g)	Chol. (mg)	Sodium (mg)	Calcium (%)	Iron (%)	Carbs (g)	Fiber (g)
2	1	0	0	0	950	0	0	0	0
0	0	0	0	0	1100	0	0	0	0
0	0	0	0	2	0	0	0	0	0
2	1	0	0	5	700	0	2	1	0
1	0	0	0	0	570	4	2	1	0
0	0	0	0	0	140	2	2	3	<1
1	0	0	0	0	450	2	2	2	0
2	0	0	0	0	550	2	2	2	0
0	0	0	0	0	920	0	0	0	0
0	0	0	0	0	910	0	0	0	0
4	19	4	0	0	1	5	4	3	2
4	1.5	0	0	0	125	4	2	9	3
3	1	0	0	0	130	4	4	12	2
3	1	0	0	0	110	2	4	13	2
4	2	0	0	0	190	4	6	19	2
4	1	0	0	0	180	2	6	18	3
4	2	0	0	0	210	4	6	19	1
4	1	0	0	0	190	6	6	18	1
3	2	1	0	0	110	0	4	17	1
2	1.5	0	0	0	230	4	4	15	1
4	1.5	0	0	0	200	10	6	20	<1

FOOD NAME	Portion Size	Calories	
Honey Wheat Berry	1 slice	100	
Honey Whole Grain	1 slice	110	
Oat & Nut	1 slice	120	
Potato	1 slice	110	
100% Multigrain	1 slice	110	
100% Whole Wheat Extra Fiber	1 slice	110	
Oroweat			
7-Grain	1 slice	100	
12-Grain	1 slice	110	
Buttermilk, Country	1 slice	100	
Healthnut	1 slice	100	
Honey Fiber Whole Grain	1 slice	80	
Jewish Rye	1 slice	80	
Oatnut	1 slice	100	
Potato, Country	1 slice	100	
Russian Rye	1 slice	80	
White, Country	1 slice	110	
Whole Grain Nut	1 slice	90	
Whole Wheat	1 slice	100	
Pepperidge Farm			
7-Grain Light	3 slices	130	
Carb Style 100% Whole Wheat	1 slice	60	
Deli Swirl	1 slice	80	
Hearty White	1 slice	120	
Honey Whole Wheat	1 slice	110	

Protein (g)	Total Fat (g)	Sat. Fat (g)	Trans Fat (g)	Chol. (mg)	Sodium (mg)	Calcium (%)	Iron (%)	Carbs (g)	Fiber (g)
4	0.5	0	0	0	220	10	6	20	1
5	1.5	0	0	0	180	10	6	19	2
4	2.5	0.5	0	0	210	10	6	20	1
4	1	0	0	0	190	10	6	20	<1
5	1.5	0	0	0	180	15	6	19	5
5	1.5	0	0	0	180	15	6	20	5
3	1	0	0	0	180	4	10	20	2
4	1.5	0	0	0	190	4	6	20	1
4	1	0	0	0	190	2	6	19	<1
4	2	0	0	0	180	2	6	18	2
4	1	0	0	0	170	15	6	18	4
3	1	0	0	0	170	0	4	14	<1
3	1.5	0.5	0	0	190	0	6	18	1
3	1	0	0	0	180	4	8	20	<1
3	1	0	0	0	200	4	4	13	<1
3	1.5	0	0	0	240	2	6	20	<1
4	1.5	0	0	0	150	4	6	18	3
4	1	0	0	0	210	6	6	19	3
7	1	0	0	0	270	6	10	26	4
5	1.5	0	0	0	170	10	4	8	3
3	1	0	0	0	180	2	4	14	1
4	1.5	0.5	0	0	250	4	6	22	1
4	2	0.5	0	0	170	4	6	20	3

Bread FOOD NAME	Portion Size	Calories	
Multigrain, Whole Grain	1 slice	120	
Pumpernickel	1 slice	80	
Sara Lee			
Classic Wheat	1 slice	70	
Country Potato	1 slice	100	
Cracked Wheat	1 slice	110	
Delightful White	2 slices	90	
Heart Healthy Multigrain	1 slice	100	
Honey Nut & Oat	1 slice	113	
Honey Wheat	1 slice	70	
Honey White	1 slice	100	
Sheepherder Country	1 slice	110	
Sourdough	1 slice	110	
Stroehmann			
Dutch Country, 12-Grain	1 slice	100	
Dutch Country, Honey Cracked Wheat	1 slice	90	
Dutch Country, Potato	1 slice	100	
Family Grains, 100% Whole Wheat	1 slice	80	
Family Grains, King White	2 slices	130	
Family Grains, Multigrain	1 slice	80	
Family Grains, Oat & Honey	1 slice	80	
Wonder			
Beefsteak, Soft Rye	1 slice	70	
Kids Sandwich	1 slice	60	
Light Wheat	2 slices	80	

Protein (g)	Total Fat (g)	Sat. Fat (g)	Trans Fat (g)	Chol. (mg)	Sodium (mg)	Calcium (%)	Iron (%)	Carbs (g)	Fiber (g)
4	2	0	0	0	200	4	4	20	3
3	1	0	0	0	190	2	6	15	1
3	1	0	0	0	150	4	na	13	2
4	1	0	0	0	210	4	na	21	1
3	1	0	0	0	210	8	na	23	2
5	1	0	0	0	240	6	na	18	4
4	1	0	0	0	180	4	na	19	2
5	1.5	0	0	0	235	8	na	21	2
2	1	0	0	0	140	2	na	14	1
3	0.5	0.5	0	0	210	4	na	22	0
4	1	0	0	0	240	4	na	21	1
4	1	0	0	0	210	0	na	22	0
3	1.5	0	0	0	150	4	6	19	1
3	1	0	0	0	170	4	6	18	1
3	1.5	0	0	0	170	2	6	19	1
4	1.5	0	0	0	140	6	4	13	2
4	1.5	0	0	0	250	6	8	25	1
3	1.5	0	0	0	110	6	4	14	2
3	1.5	0	0	0	150	6	4	14	2
2	1	0	0	0	180	2	4	14	<1
2	0.5	0	0	0	115	20	8	12	2
5	0.5	0	0	0	240	15	8	18	5

Bread – Broccoli, fresh, boiled, chopped FOOD NAME	Portion Size	Calories	
Stone Ground 100% Whole Wheat	1 slice	80	
Whole Grain White	2 slices	130	
BREAD, Frozen (Pepperidge Farm)			
Garlic	2.5" slice	160	
Texas Toast, Garlic	1 slice	150	
Texas Toast, Mozzarella & Monterey Jack	1 slice	160	
BREADCRUMBS			
Devonsheer, Plain	⅛ c	110	
Progresso, Plain	¼ c	110	
Progresso, Garlic & Herb	¼ c	110	
Progresso, Italian Style	¼ c	110	
BROCCOLI, fresh, boiled, chopped	½ c	27	
Frozen, Birds Eye			
Chopped	¾ c	30	
Florets	1 c	30	
Tender Cuts	1 c	30	
w/ Cheese Sauce	½ c	90	
w/ Beans, Peppers, Onion	1 c	30	
w/ Corn & Peppers	¾ c	60	
w/ Peppers, Onion, Mushrooms	1 c	30	
w/ Cauliflower & Peppers	1 c	25	
Frozen, Green Giant			
Spears in Butter	4 oz	50	
w/ Cauliflower, Carrots, Cheese	⅔ c	60	
w/ Cheese	⅔ c	60	

Protein (g)	Total Fat (g)	Sat. Fat (g)	Trans Fat (g)	Chol. (mg)	Sodium (mg)	Calcium (%)	Iron (%)	Carbs (g)	Fiber (g)
4	1	0	0	0	170	4	4	14	2
6	2	0.5	0	0	240	35	15	25	4
5	6	1.5	na	0	270	2	8	23	2
3	7	2	3	0	190	0	6	18	2
5	7	1.5	1	<5	250	6	6	20	<1
4	1.5	0	0	0	200	na	na	19	1
4	1.5	0.5	0	0	220	4	8	20	1
4	1.5	0.5	0	0	540	4	8	20	1
4	1.5	0.5	0	0	470	4	8	20	1
2	0	0	0	0	32	3	3	6	3
1	0	0	0	0	20	2	0	4	2
1	0	0	0	0	20	2	0	4	2
1	0	0	0	0	20	2	0	4	2
3	5	3	0	5	490	6	2	8	1
1	0	0	0	0	10	2	2	5	2
2	1	0	0	0	10	2	2	11	1
1	0	0	0	0	15	2	2	4	1
1	0	0	0	0	20	2	2	3	1
3	2	1	0	<5	330	0	0	6	2
2	2.5	1	0	<5	500	4	0	8	2
2	2.5	1	0	<5	520	4	0	7	2

FOOD NAME	Portion Size	Calories	
w/ Three Cheese Sauce	⅔ c	50	
w/ Zesty Cheese	¾ c	60	
BRUSSELS SPROUTS, fresh, boiled	½ c	28	
Birds Eye, frozen	10 pc	45	
Birds Eye, w/Cauliflower & Carrots	1 c	40	
Green Giant, w/Butter Sauce	½ c	70	
BULGUR, cooked	1 c	151	
BUTTER, regular, salted	1 Tbs	100	
Whipped, salted	1 Tbs	66	
BUTTERMILK, low-fat	1 c	98	
CABBAGE			
Green, raw, shredded	½ c	8	
Green, boiled, no salt, shredded	½ c	16	
Napa, cooked	1 c	13	
Red, raw, chopped	1 c	28	
Red, boiled, shredded	1 c	44	
Savoy, raw, shredded	1 c	19	
Savoy, boiled, shredded	1 c	35	
CAKE, bakery-type			
Entenmann's, All-Butter Loaf	⅙ cake	220	
Entenmann's, Caramel Mocha	⅙ cake	260	
Entenmann's, Cinnamon Crumb	⅑ cake	320	
Entenmann's, Coffee House Crunch	⅙ cake	290	
Entenmann's, Filled Chocolate Chip Crumb	⅑ cake	390	
Entenmann's, French Crumb	⅛ cake	210	

Protein (g)	Total Fat (g)	Sat. Fat (g)	Trans Fat (g)	Chol. (mg)	Sodium (mg)	Calcium (%)	Iron (%)	Carbs (g)	Fiber (g)
2	2	0.5	0.5	<5	510	4	2	7	2
2	2	0.5	0	<5	470	4	0	8	1
2	0	0	0	0	16	3	5	6	2
3	0	0	0	0	15	2	4	8	3
2	0	0	0	0	35	2	2	7	2
4	1	0.5	0	<5	320	2	2	10	3
6	0	0	0	0	9	2	10	34	8
0	11	7	0	0	81	30	0	0	0
0	8	5	0	20	76	0	0	0	0
8	2	1	0	10	257	28	1	12	0
0	0	0	0	0	8	2	1	2	1
1	0	0	0	0	6	2	1	3	1
1	0	0	0	0	12	3	4	2	0
1	0	0	0	0	24	4	4	7	2
2	0	0	0	0	12	6	6	10	4
1	0	0	0	0	20	2	2	4	2
3	0	0	0	0	35	4	3	8	4
3	9	6	0	70	280	2	0	31	0
2	12	5	0	10	200	6	4	36	<1
3	14	5	0	45	210	15	2	45	<1
3	14	5	0	35	190	4	6	39	1
3	1	8	0	35	210	4	6	49	1
2	10	5	0	50	230	0	2	29	<1

Cake, bakery-type – Cake, boxed (mix only unless noted) FOOD NAME	Portion Size	Calories	
Entenmann's, Louisiana Crumb	1/9 cake	330	
Entenmann's Pina Colada	1/6 cake	290	
CAKE, boxed (mix only unless noted)			
Betty Crocker			
Angel Food Confetti	1/12 cake	150	
Angel Food White	1/12 cake	140	
Brownie, Fudge, Chewy	1/20 pkg	110	
Brownie, Fudge, Low-Fat, prep	1/18 pkg	130	
Brownie, Supreme, Frosted	1/20 pkg	150	
Brownie, Supreme, Peanut Butter	1/20 pkg	130	
Brownie, Supreme, Turtle	1/20 pkg	120	
Complete Desserts, Hot Fudge Cake	1/6 pkg	430	
Gingerbread Cake & Cookie Mix	1/8 pkg	210	
Pineapple Upside Down Cake	1/6 cake	350	
Pound Cake	1/8 cake	240	
Quick Bread, Banana	1/12 cake	130	
Quick Bread, Cinnamon Streusel	1/14 cake	160	
Quick bread, Cranberry Orange	1/12 cake	150	
Quick bread, Lemon Poppy Seed	1/12 cake	130	
SuperMoist			
Butter Pecan	1/12 cake	170	
Butter Recipe Chocolate	1/12 cake	170	
Carrot	1/12 cake	200	
Chocolate Fudge	1/12 cake	170	
Cinnamon Swirl	1/12 cake	200	

Protein (g)	Total Fat (g)	Sat. Fat (g)	Trans Fat (g)	Chol. (mg)	Sodium (mg)	Calcium (%)	Iron (%)	Carbs (g)	Fiber (g)
3	14	4	0	45	300	15	2	49	<1
2	15	7	0	25	170	4	0	36	0
3	0	0	0	0	320	6	na	34	na
3	0	0	0	0	320	6	na	32	na
1	1.5	0.5	0.5	0	100	2	4	24	na
2	2.5	1	0.5	0	115	na	6	27	na
1	3	1	1	0	125	2	6	30	1
2	3	2	0.5	0	100	2	4	23	na
1	2.5	0.5	0	0	95	2	4	23	na
5	13	5	1	5	620	4	10	75	na
2	5	1.5	1.5	0	360	6	10	39	na
2	9	2.5	3	0	280	4	4	65	na
2	7	2.5	1.5	0	190	4	4	45	na
2	2.5	0.5	1	0	190	na	4	25	na
2	4	1	1	0	150	2	4	28	na
2	3	0.5	0.5	0	170	na	2	29	na
2	2.5	0.5	0.5	0	190	0	4	25	na
1	3	1.5	1	0	270	6	4	35	na
2	3	1.5	0.5	0	340	4	10	35	2
2	3	1	1	0	350	10	4	42	na
2	3	1	0.5	0	340	4	6	35	1
2	3.5	1	1	0	290	8	6	42	na

Cake, boxed (mix only unless noted) – Cake, Snack FOOD NAME	Portion Size	Calories	
French Vanilla	1/12 cake	170	
German Chocolate	1/12 cake	170	
Lemon	1/12 cake	170	
Pineapple	1/12 cake	170	
Rainbow Chip	1/10 cake	210	
Spice	1/12 cake	170	
Strawberry	1/12 cake	170	
Triple Chocolate Fudge	1/12 cake	180	
Yellow	1/12 cake	170	
CAKE, Frozen			
Pepperidge Farm, Coconut	1/8 cake	250	
Pepperidge Farm, Chocolate Fudge	1/8 cake	250	
Pepperidge Farm, Chocolate Fudge Stripe	1/8 cake	250	
Pepperidge Farm, Vanilla	1/8 cake	250	
CAKE, Snack			
Drake's, Coffee Cake	2	280	
Drake's, Devil Dogs	1	170	
Drake's, Devil Dogs, Reduced Fat	1	160	
Drake's, Funny Bones, Peanut Butter	2	310	
Drake's, Yodels	2	280	
Hostess, Chocolate Cupcakes	1	180	
Hostess, Ho Hos, Caramel	3 cakes	380	
Hostess, Twinkies	1	150	
Tastykake			
Chocolate Cupcakes, single serve	3 cakes	310	

Protein (g)	Total Fat (g)	Sat. Fat (g)	Trans Fat (g)	Chol. (mg)	Sodium (mg)	Calcium (%)	Iron (%)	Carbs (g)	Fiber (g)
1	3	1.5	1	0	280	6	4	35	na
2	3	1	0.5	0	330	4	4	35	1
1	3	1.5	1	0	280	6	4	35	na
1	3	1.5	1	0	280	6	4	35	na
2	4.5	1.5	1	0	320	6	4	41	na
1	3.5	1.5	1	0	280	8	4	35	na
1	3	1.5	1	0	270	6	4	35	na
2	4	2	0.5	0	320	4	6	34	na
1	3	1.5	1	0	280	6	4	35	na
2	11	3	3	25	115	0	0	35	<1
3	11	3	3.5	30	160	0	6	31	1
2	13	3	3.5	25	140	0	6	31	1
2	11	2.5	3.5	25	120	0	0	35	<1
3	12	2.5	2.5	15	200	2	8	40	1
2	7	2	2	0	150	0	6	26	1
2	4	1	1	8	180	2	6	29	1
5	16	8	1.5	0	270	2	6	38	2
2	14	8	2	20	160	2	4	36	1
2	6	2.5	0	5	290	10	6	30	<1
3	18	12	1.5	25	210	2	6	53	2
1	4.5	2.5	0	20	220	2	na	27	0
4	10	3	2	10	390	2	10	55	3

Cake, Snack – Candy

FOOD NAME	Portion Size	Calories	
Chocolate Cupcakes, Cream Filled, single serve	3 cakes	370	
Chocolate Junior, single serve	1	340	
Coconut Junior, single serve	1	340	
Fudge Nut Brownies	½	150	
Glazed Honey Bun, family pack	1	330	
Kandy Kake, Boston Kreme	2 cakes	150	
Kandy Kake, Mint	2 cakes	170	
Kreamies, Banana	1	170	
Krimpets, Butterscotch	2 cakes	210	
Krimpets, Jelly	2 cakes	180	
Raspberry Koffee Kake, low-fat	2 cakes	170	
Snowballs	1	210	
CANDY			
Almond Joy (Hershey's)	45 g	220	
Bit-O-Honey (Nestlé)	6 pc	160	
Caramello	6 blocks	200	
Chocolate bar, Dairy Milk (Cadbury)	10 blocks	220	
Chocolate bar, Fruit & Nut (Cadbury)	10 blocks	200	
Chocolate bar (Hershey's)	43 g	230	
Chocolate bar, pure dark (Hershey's)	3 blocks	210	
Chocolate bar, milk w/almonds	41 g	230	
Chocolate bar, w/caramel (Hershey's 'N' More)	25 g	110	
5th Avenue	56 g	280	

Protein (g)	Total Fat (g)	Sat. Fat (g)	Trans Fat (g)	Chol. (mg)	Sodium (mg)	Calcium (%)	Iron (%)	Carbs (g)	Fiber (g)
4	14	3.5	3	15	370	4	8	58	1
4	12	3.5	2.5	75	180	2	10	54	0
4	12	2.5	0	75	180	2	10	54	0
2	7	1.5	0	10	71	0	na	27	0
3	18	4	7	0	220	8	8	38	<1
1	9	4.5	0	10	65	2	na	24	0
2	9	5	0	0	0	2	na	24	0
1	8	2	2	5	100	2	2	25	0
2	6	2	1	30	170	2	2	37	0
2	4	1	0	60	220	2	6	34	0
2	2.5	0.5	0	0	170	2	na	35	0
2	7	2.5	0	18	200	0	4	36	0
2	12	8	0	0	65	2	2	27	2
1	3	2	0	0	120	2	1	32	0
3	9	6	0	10	50	9	2	27	<1
3	12	8	0	10	45	10	2	24	<1
3	10	5	0	5	30	8	2	25	1
3	13	9	0	10	40	8	2	25	1
3	13	8	0	<5	5	2	20	20	4
4	14	6	0	5	30	8	2	22	2
<1	5	4	0	0	50	0	0	15	0
4	14	5	0	0	140	2	2	5	2

Candy		
FOOD NAME	Portion Size	Calories
Goobers	10 pc	51
Heath Toffee Bar	39 g	220
Kisses (Hershey's)	9 pc	230
Kisses, Hugs	9 pc	210
Kisses w/peanut butter	9 pc	230
Kit Kat	1 4-pc	220
Kit Kat, white	1 4-pc	220
Krackel	41 g	210
Milk Duds	13 pc	180
M&M's	1.69 oz	240
M&M's, peanut	1.74 oz	250
M&M's, Almond	1.31 oz	200
Milky Way	2.05 oz	260
Milky Way Midnight	1.76 oz	220
Mounds	49 g	240
Mr. Goodbar	49 g	270
Pay Day	52 g	250
Raisinets	1 oz	116
Reese's NutRageous	51 g	280
Reese's peanut butter & white chocolate	42 g	230
Reese's Pieces	43 g	220
Rolo	48 g	210
S'mores	46 g	230
Skor	39 g	210
Symphony, Milk Chocolate	42 g	230

Protein (g)	Total Fat (g)	Sat. Fat (g)	Trans Fat (g)	Chol. (mg)	Sodium (mg)	Calcium (%)	Iron (%)	Carbs (g)	Fiber (g)
1	3	1	0	1	4	1	1	5	1
1	13	7	0	10	140	2	0	24	0
3	13	8	0	10	35	8	2	24	1
3	12	7	0	10	45	10	0	23	0
4	14	7	0	5	105	4	2	21	1
3	11	7	0	<5	25	4	2	27	<1
3	12	8	0	5	45	8	0	26	0
2	10	6	0	<5	50	4	2	28	<1
1	7	3.5	0	0	85	4	0	28	0
2	10	6	0	5	30	4	2	34	1
5	13	5	0	5	25	4	2	30	2
3	11	3.5	0	5	15	4	2	21	2
2	10	7	0	5	95	6	0	41	1
2	8	5	0	5	90	2	2	36	1
2	13	10	0	0	70	0	4	29	2
5	16	7	0	5	20	4	2	27	2
6	13	2.5	0	0	160	2	2	28	2
1	4	2	0	1	10	3	2	20	0
6	16	5	0	0	105	2	2	27	2
5	13	4.5	0	<5	150	6	0	22	1
5	11	7	0	0	80	2	0	26	1
2	9	7	0	5	85	6	0	31	0
2	11	6	0	<5	65	4	2	31	<1
1	12	7	0	15	120	2	0	24	<1
4	13	8	0	10	40	10	2	24	<1

FOOD NAME	Portion Size	Calories	
Take 5	42 g	210	
Tootsie Roll	6 pc	155	
Twix	1 oz	155	
Twizzlers, Strawberry	2.5 oz	249	
Whoppers	21 g	100	
York Peppermint Patty	39 g	160	
CANTALOUPE, raw	½ med	94	
CARROTS			
Raw, large	1 7-8.5"	30	
Cooked, no salt, sliced	½ c	27	
Birds Eye, frozen, whole baby	⅔ c	35	
Birds Eye, frozen, sliced	⅔ c	35	
Del Monte canned	½ c	35	
Del Monte canned, 'honey glazed	½ c	70	
CARROT JUICE, Odwalla	8 oz	70	
Hain w/ Lutein	8 oz	80	
CASABA MELON, raw, cubes	1 c	48	
CASHEWS, dry roast, no salt	1 oz	162	
CASHEW BUTTER, Maranatha	2 Tbs	190	
CAULIFLOWER, raw	1 c	25	
Boiled, no salt	1 c	28	
Birds Eye, Frozen, Florets	4 pc	25	
Birds Eye, Cauliflower & Garlic Sauce	1¼ c	60	
Bird's Eye, Cauliflower, Carrots &			
Snow Pea Pods	1 c	30	

Protein (g)	Total Fat (g)	Sat. Fat (g)	Trans Fat (g)	Chol. (mg)	Sodium (mg)	Calcium (%)	Iron (%)	Carbs (g)	Fiber (g)
4	10	5	0	<5	180	2	2	26	1
1	1	0	0	1	18	1	2	35	0
2	9	1	0	2	75	4	2	16	1
2	2	0	0	0	204	0	2	57	0
<1	3.5	3	0	0	70	4	0	16	0
<1	3	1.5	0	0	10	0	2	32	<1
3	<1	0	0	0	44	3	3	22	3
1	0	0	0	0	50	2	1	7	2
1	0	0	0	0	45	2	1	6	2
0	0	0	0	0	60	2	0	7	2
0	0	0	0	0	55	2	0	7	2
0	0	0	0	0	300	2	2	8	3
1	0	0	0	0	440	4	2	18	1
2	0	0	0	0	160	4	4	15	1
2	0.5	0	0	0	65	15	4	16	0
2	0	0	0	0	15	2	3	11	2
4	13	3	0	0	5	1	9	9	1
5	15	3	0	0	5	2	10	11	2
2	0	0	0	0	30	2	2	5	3
1	0	0	0	0	9	1	1	3	2
1	0	0	0	0	25	0	0	4	1
2	4	1	0	0	460	4	2	6	2
1	0	0	0	0	35	2	2	6	2

FOOD NAME	Portion Size	Calories	
Green Giant, Cauliflower & Cheese Sauce	½ c	50	
Green Giant, Cauliflower & Three cheese sauce, prep	½ c	45	
CAVIAR, red & black	1 oz	71	
CELERY, raw, stalk	⅞"	6	
Chopped	1 c	14	
CEREAL, cold/dry, ready-to-eat			
Arrowhead Mills			
Amaranth Flakes	1 c	140	
Bran Flakes	1 c	110	
Kamut Flakes	1 c	120	
Multigrain Flakes	1 c	170	
Organic Nature O's	1 c	130	
Puffed Corn	1 c	60	
Puffed Millet	1 c	60	
Rice Flakes, Sweetened	1 c	180	
Sweetened Shredded Wheat	1 c	200	
Barbara's Bakery			
Alpen, Original	⅔ c	200	
Brown Rice Crisps	1 c	120	
Honey Nut O's, Organic	¾ c	120	
Organic Wild Puffs, Caramel	¾ c	110	
Puffins, Original	¾ c	90	
Puffins, Peanut Butter	¾ c	110	
Shredded Oats	1¼ c	220	

Protein (g)	Total Fat (g)	Sat. Fat (g)	Trans Fat (g)	Chol. (mg)	Sodium (mg)	Calcium (%)	Iron (%)	Carbs (g)	Fiber (g)
2	2.5	1	0	0	410	4	2	6	1
2	2	0.5	0	5	300	4	0	6	1
7	5	1	0	166	424	8	19	1	0
0	0	0	0	0	32	2	0	1	1
1	0	0	0	0	81	4	1	3	2
4	2	0	0	0	0	2	6	26	3
4	1	0	0	0	85	2	6	22	5
4	1	0.5	0	0	70	2	8	25	2
5	2	0	0	0	180	2	10	33	3
4	2	0.5	0	0	0	0	6	25	2
2	1	0	0	0	5	0	2	12	2
2	0.5	0	0	0	0	0	2	11	1
3	1	0	0	0	190	0	4	40	1
5	1	0	0	0	5	2	8	42	5
6	3	0	0	0	30	6	45	41	4
2	1	0	0	0	125	0	2	25	1
3	2	0	0	0	80	8	45	24	2
2	1	0	0	0	160	4	45	25	<1
2	1	0	0	0	190	0	2	23	5
3	2	0.5	0	0	230	2	6	23	2
6	2.5	0.5	0	0	260	2	10	46	5

Cereal, cold/dry, ready-to-eat

FOOD NAME	Portion Size	Calories
Soy Essence	¾ c	110
General Mills		
Apple Cinnamon Cheerios	¾ c	120
Cheerios	1 c	110
Cheerios, Honey Nut	¾ c	110
Cheerios, Multigrain	1 c	110
Basic 4	1 c	202
Cinnamon Toast Crunch	¾ c	127
Cocoa Puffs	1 c	117
Corn Chex	1 c	112
Corn Flakes	1 c	111
Fiber One	½ c	60
Frosted Wheaties	¾ c	112
Golden Grahams	¾ c	112
Kix	1¼ c	110
Lucky Charms	¾ c	110
Nature Valley Low-Fat Fruit Granola	⅔ c	212
Oatmeal Crisp w/ Almonds	1 c	218
Oatmeal Raisin Crisp	1 c	204
Rice Chex	1¼ c	117
Total, Whole grain	¾ c	97
Total, Corn Flakes	1⅓ c	112
Trix	1 c	117
Wheaties	¾ c	100
Health Valley		

Protein (g)	Total Fat (g)	Sat. Fat (g)	Trans Fat (g)	Chol. (mg)	Sodium (mg)	Calcium (%)	Iron (%)	Carbs (g)	Fiber (g)
4	0.5	0	0	0	115	2	8	25	5
2	1.5	0	0	0	120	10	25	25	1
3	2	0	0	0	210	10	45	22	3
3	1.5	0	0	0	190	10	25	22	2
2	1	0	0	0	200	10	100	23	3
4	3	0	0	0	316	20	20	42	3
2	3	1	0	0	206	10	26	24	1
1	1	0	0	0	171	10	25	26	1
2	0	0	0	0	288	10	50	26	1
2	0	0	0	0	263	25	45	26	1
2	1	0	0	0	105	10	25	25	14
2	0	0	0	0	204	10	45	27	1
2	1	0	0	0	210	10	25	25	1
2	1	0	0	0	210	15	45	26	1
2	1	0	0	0	190	10	25	22	1
4	3	0	0	0	207	2	6	44	3
6	5	1	0	0	236	2	25	42	4
5	2	0	0	0	216	2	25	45	4
2	0	0	0	0	292	10	52	27	0
3	1	0	0	0	192	119	124	22	3
2	0	0	0	0	209	100	100	26	1
1	1	0	0	0	194	10	25	27	1
3	0.5	0	0	0	180	2	45	22	3

Cereal, cold/dry, ready-to-eat FOOD NAME	Portion Size	Calories	
Corn Crunch-Ems	1 c	110	
Date Almond Granola, low-fat	⅔ c	180	
Heart Wise	1 c	200	
Organic Amaranth Flakes	¾ c	100	
Organic Blue Corn Flakes	¾ c	100	
Organic Oat Bran Flakes w/ Raisins	¾ c	110	
Original Soy Flakes	1¼ c	190	
Raisin Cinnamon Granola, low-fat	⅔ c	180	
Slender	1 c	180	
Kashi			
Go Lean	¾ c	114	
Good Friends	¾ c	95	
Heart to Heart	¾ c	115	
Medley	¾ c	113	
Organic Promise, Autumn Wheat	1 c	181	
Organic Promise, Cranberry	1 c	92	
Organic Promise, Strawberry Fields	1 c	111	
Seven in the Morning	1 c	207	
Kellogg's			
All-Bran Buds	⅓ c	70	
Apple Jacks	1 c	130	
Cocoa Krispies	¾ c	120	
Complete Oat Bran Flakes	¾ c	110	
Corn Flakes	1 c	101	
Corn Pops	1 c	117	

Protein (g)	Total Fat (g)	Sat. Fat (g)	Trans Fat (g)	Chol. (mg)	Sodium (mg)	Calcium (%)	Iron (%)	Carbs (g)	Fiber (g)
4	0	0	0	0	160	na	na	27	2
6	1	0	0	0	90	2	8	43	6
11	3	0	0	0	120	30	50	36	5
3	0	0	0	0	90	0	4	24	4
3	0	0	0	0	10	0	4	24	3
3	0	0	0	0	90	0	4	26	4
13	1.5	0	0	0	190	4	15	35	5
5	1	0	0	0	90	2	8	43	6
5	1.5	0	0	0	130	30	50	35	4
10	1	0	0	0	66	6	11	23	8
3	1	9	9	9	73	1	5	25	7
4	2	0	0	0	1	2	12	25	5
3	1	0	0	0	74	1	4	26	3
5	1	0	0	0	2	3	9	45	8
2	1	0	0	0	21	0	2	26	3
3	0	0	0	0	200	1	3	28	1
7	2	0	0	0	260	2	74	47	7
2	1	0	0	0	200	0	25	24	13
1	0.5	0	0	0	150	0	25	30	1
1	1	0.5	0	0	190	4	25	27	1
3	1	0	0	0	210	0	100	23	4
2	0	0	0	0	202	0	45	24	1
1	0	0	0	0	120	1	11	28	0

Cereal, cold/dry, ready-to-eat

FOOD NAME	Portion Size	Calories	
Cracklin' Oat Bran	¾ c	220	
Froot Loops	1 c	120	
Frosted Flakes	¾ c	120	
Frosted Mini Wheats, Bite-Size Biscuits	24 pc	200	
Just Right Fruit & Nut	¾ c	200	
Low-Fat Granola w/ Raisins	⅔ c	201	
Mueslix	⅔ c	200	
Product 19	1 c	100	
Puffed Wheat	1 oz	94	
Raisin Bran	1 c	190	
Rice Krispies	1¼ c	120	
Rice Krispies Treat Cereal	¾ c	120	
Smart Start Antioxidants	1 c	190	
Smart Start Healthy Heart Maple			
Brown Sugar	1¼ c	230	
Special K	1 c	110	
Malt-O-Meal			
Apple-Cinnamon Toasty O's	¾ c	120	
Coco Roos	¾ c	120	
Colossal Crunch	¾ c	120	
Crispy Rice	1¼ c	130	
Frosted Flakes	¾ c	120	
Frosted Mini Spooners	1 c	190	
Honey Nut Toasty O's	1 c	110	
Marshmallow Mateys	1 c	120	

Protein (g)	Total Fat (g)	Sat. Fat (g)	Trans Fat (g)	Chol. (mg)	Sodium (mg)	Calcium (%)	Iron (%)	Carbs (g)	Fiber (g)
4	7	3	0	0	150	2	10	35	6
1	1	0.5	0	0	150	0	25	28	1
1	0	0	0	0	150	0	25	28	1
6	1	0	0	0	5	2	90	48	6
4	2	0	0	0	240	2	50	43	3
4	3	1	0	0	135	2	9	44	3
5	3	0	0	0	170	2	25	40	4
2	0	0	0	0	210	0	100	25	1
3	0	0	0	0	1	1	0	23	3
5	1.5	0	0	0	360	2	25	45	7
2	0	0	0	0	320	0	10	29	0
1	1.5	0	0	0	170	0	10	26	0
3	0.5	0	0	0	280	0	100	43	3
7	3	0.5	0	0	140	2	25	46	5
7	0	0	0	0	220	0	45	22	<1
2	1.5	0	0	0	160	10	25	25	2
1	1.5	0	0	0	135	10	25	26	<1
1	1.5	0	0	0	230	0	25	26	0
2	0	0	0	0	300	0	50	29	0
2	0	0	0	0	180	0	25	28	1
5	1	0	0	0	10	0	90	45	6
2	1.5	0	0	0	210	10	25	24	2
2	1	0	0	0	200	10	25	25	1

Cereal, cold/dry, ready-to-eat FOOD NAME	Portion Size	Calories	
Raisin Bran	1 c	220	
Tootie Fruities	1 c	130	
Post			
Alpha Bits	1 oz	110	
Banana Nut Crunch	2 oz	240	
Blueberry Morning Selects	2 oz	230	
Bran Flakes	1 oz	100	
Cocoa Pebbles	1 oz	110	
Cranberry Almond Crunch Selects	2 oz	220	
Fruit & Bran	2 oz	200	
Golden Crisp	1 oz	110	
Grape Nuts	2 oz	200	
Grape Nut Flakes	1 oz	110	
Great Grains Crunchy Pecans Selects	2 oz	220	
Honey Bunches of Oats, Honey Roasted	1 c	120	
Honey Bunches of Oats, Strawberry	1 oz	120	
Honeycomb	1 oz	120	
Maple Pecan Crunch Selects	2 oz	220	
Oreo O's	1 oz	110	
Quaker			
Life, Cinnamon	¾ c	120	
Life, Honey graham	¾ c	120	
Life, Original	¾ c	120	
Mother's Peanut Butter Bumpers	1 c	130	
Mother's Toasted Oat Bran	¾ c	120	

Protein (g)	Total Fat (g)	Sat. Fat (g)	Trans Fat (g)	Chol. (mg)	Sodium (mg)	Calcium (%)	Iron (%)	Carbs (g)	Fiber (g)
5	1	0	0	0	350	2	25	47	7
2	1	0	0	0	150	10	25	28	1
4	2	0	0	0	190	10	45	22	3
5	6	0.5	0	0	250	2	90	44	5
4	3	0	0	0	250	0	10	48	3
3	0.5	0	0	0	220	0	45	24	3
1	1.5	1	0	0	190	0	10	26	3
4	3	0	0	0	190	0	10	44	3
4	3	0	0	0	260	2	30	42	6
2	0	0	0	0	25	0	10	25	1
7	1	0	0	0	310	2	90	47	6
3	1	0	0	0	120	0	45	24	3
5	6	1	0	0	200	0	50	38	4
2	1.5	0	0	0	170	0	45	25	2
2	2	0	0	0	150	0	45	26	1
2	1	0	0	0	170	0	15	28	3
5	6	1	0	0	200	0	50	38	4
1	2	0.5	0	0	90	0	10	22	1
3	1.5	0	0	0	150	10	40	25	2
3	1.5	0	0	0	160	10	50	25	2
3	1.5	0	0	0	160	10	45	25	2
3	2.5	0.5	0	0	270	2	6	26	1
4	1.5	0	0	0	200	2	6	24	3

FOOD NAME	Portion Size	Calories	
CEREALS, hot			
Arrowhead Mills			
4 Grains Plus Flax	¼ c	140	
Bear Mush	¼ c	150	
Bits O Barley	¼ c	160	
Instant Maple Apple Spice	1 pkt	140	
Instant Oatmeal, Original	1 pkt	110	
Oat Flakes	⅓ c	130	
Rice and Shine	¼ c	150	
Yellow Corn Grits	¼ c	130	
Cream of Wheat			
Apple & Cinnamon Instant	1 pkt	130	
Cinnamon Swirl	1 pkt	130	
Maple Brown Sugar	1 pkt	120	
Quaker			
Instant, Apples & Cinnamon	1 pkt	130	
Instant, Maple & Brown Sugar	1 pkt	160	
Multigrain Hot Cereal	½ c	130	
Nutrition for Women, Golden Brown Sugar	1 pkt	160	
Nutrition for Women, Vanilla Cinnamon	1 pkt	160	
Oatmeal, Express Baked Apple	1 c	200	
Oatmeal, Express Cinnamon Roll	1 c	210	
Quick Oats	½ c	150	
CEREAL BARS			
Barbara's Bakery			

Cereals, hot – Cereal Bars

Protein (g)	Total Fat (g)	Sat. Fat (g)	Trans Fat (g)	Chol. (mg)	Sodium (mg)	Calcium (%)	Iron (%)	Carbs (g)	Fiber (g)
4	2	0	0	0	45	2	6	26	3
5	1	0	0	0	0	15	4	32	2
4	1	0	0	0	0	0	2	34	6
4	2	0	0	0	45	2	6	26	3
4	2	0	0	0	0	0	4	19	2
5	2	0.5	0	0	0	2	8	23	4
3	1	0	0	0	0	0	4	32	2
3	0	0	0	0	0	0	2	30	1
2	0	0	0	0	160	20	45	29	1
2	0	0	0	0	170	20	45	28	1
2	0	0	0	0	140	20	45	27	1
3	1.5	0.5	0	0	170	10	20	27	3
4	2	0	0	0	270	10	20	33	3
5	1	0	0	0	0	0	6	29	5
6	2.5	0.5	0	0	330	50	35	32	3
5	2	0.5	0	0	290	50	35	32	3
4	2.5	0.5	0	0	320	10	20	42	4
5	3.5	0.5	0	0	250	10	20	41	3
5	3	0.5	0	0	0	0	10	27	4

FOOD NAME	Portion Size	Calories	
Fruit & Yogurt Bars, Apple Cinnamon	1	150	
Fruit & Yogurt Bars, Blueberry Apple	1	150	
Fruit & Yogurt bars, Cherry Apple	1	150	
Granola, Carob Chip	1	80	
Granola, Cinnamon & Raisin	1	80	
Granola, Oats & Honey	1	80	
Granola, Peanut Butter	1	80	
Multigrain, Apple Cinnamon	1	120	
Multigrain, Cherry	1	120	
Puffins Cereal & Milk Bars, Blueberry	1	140	
Puffins, Cereal & Milk Bars, French Toast	1	130	
Puffins, Cereal & Milk Bars, Peanut Butter Chocolate Chip	1	140	
Cascadian Farm			
Granola, Chocolate Chip	1	140	
Granola, Fruit & Nut	1	140	
Granola, Harvest Berries	1	130	
Granola, Multigrain	1	130	
Health Valley			
Apple Cobbler	1	130	
Apricot Fruit Bar, fat-free	1	140	
Café Creations, Cinnamon Danish Bar	1	130	
Café Creations, Chocolate Raspberry	1	130	
Fig Cobbler Cereal Bar	1		
Moist & Chewy Dutch Apple Granola	1	100	

Protein (g)	Total Fat (g)	Sat. Fat (g)	Trans Fat (g)	Chol. (mg)	Sodium (mg)	Calcium (%)	Iron (%)	Carbs (g)	Fiber (g)
3	3	0	0	0	125	25	10	28	1
3	3	0	0	0	125	25	10	29	1
3	3	0	0	0	125	25	10	29	1
2	2	0	0	0	0	2	2	15	<1
2	2	0	0	0	0	2	2	14	<1
2	2	0	0	0	0	2	2	14	<1
2	3	0	0	0	0	0	2	13	<1
1	1.5	0	0	0	65	0	2	25	2
1	1.5	0	0	0	65	0	2	25	2
5	1.5	1	0	0	85	30	30	24	3
6	1.5	1	0	0	100	30	30	24	3
0	3.5	1.5	0	0	160	30	30	20	3
2	3	1	0	0	125	0	6	25	1
2	4	0.5	0	0	110	0	2	24	1
2	2	0	0	0	130	0	0	27	1
2	2	0	0	0	150	0	0	27	1
2	2	0	0	0	50	na	4	27	1
2	0	0	0	0	10	2	6	35	3
2	2.5	0	0	0	80	2	4	27	2
1	3	0	0	0	50	2	4	27	2
2	1	0	0	0	15	na	4	22	2

Cereal Bars – Cheese		
FOOD NAME	Portion Size	Calories
Peanut Butter & Grape Bar	1	130
Raspberry Granola Bar, f-f	1	140
Strawberry Cobbler Cereal Bar	1	130
Kellogg's		
All-Bran Brown Sugar Cinnamon Bar	1	130
Cocoa Krispies Cereal & Milk Bar	1	100
Nutri-Grain, Apple Cinnamon	1	140
Nutri-Grain, Cherry	1	140
Nutri-Grain, Mixed Berry	1	140
Nutri-Grain, Muffin Bar, Banana	1	170
Nutri-Grain, Muffin Bar, Cinnamon & Raisin	1	170
Nutri-Grain, Yogurt Bar, Strawberry	1	140
Nature Valley		
Apple Crisp	1	140
Banana Nut	1	90
Maple Brown Sugar	1	90
Oats & Honey	1	90
Peanut Butter	1	89
Pecan Crunch	1	90
Roasted Almond	1	90
Quaker		
Breakfast Bar, Strawberry	1	130
Cranberry Orange Muffin	1	130
Iced Raspberry	1	130
CHEESE		

Protein (g)	Total Fat (g)	Sat. Fat (g)	Trans Fat (g)	Chol. (mg)	Sodium (mg)	Calcium (%)	Iron (%)	Carbs (g)	Fiber (g)
2	2.5	0	0	0	140	2	10	26	1
2	0	0	0	0	10	2	6	35	3
2	2	0	0	0	50	na	4	27	1
2	3	0.5	0	0	180	0	10	27	5
1	2.5	2	0	0	80	10	8	17	0
1	3	0.5	0	0	105	20	10	26	1
1	3	0.5	0	0	100	20	10	26	<1
1	3	0.5	0	0	105	20	10	26	<1
3	4	0.5	0	0	110	0	10	30	1
2	4	0.5	0	0	100	0	10	32	1
1	3	0.5	0	0	105	20	10	26	1
2	3.5	2	0	0	130	10	2	26	1
2	3.5	0.5	0	0	80	0	2	14	1
2	3	0	0	0	80	na	2	15	1
2	3	0	0	0	80	na	2	15	1
2	3.5	0	0	0	95	na	2	15	1
2	3.5	0.5	0	0	85	na	2	14	1
2	3.5	0.5	0	0	90	0	2	14	1
1	2.5	0.5	0	0	110	20	2	27	1
1	2.5	0.5	0	0	140	20	2	26	1
1	2.5	0.5	0.5	0	100	20	2	26	1

Cheese FOOD NAME	Portion Size	Calories	
American (Alpine Lace)	1 slice	90	
American, 2% milk, singles (Kraft)	1 slice	50	
American, singles (Kraft)	1 slice	60	
American, Deli Delux (Kraft)	1 slice	80	
American (Land-O-Lakes)	1 oz	110	
American, burger, deli style (Sargento)	1 slice	70	
Blue cheese, natural crumbled (Sargento)	¼ c	100	
Blue Cheese, crumbles (Organic Valley)	1 oz	100	
Camembert	1 oz	85	
Cheddar, reduced fat (Alpine Lace)	1 slice	90	
Cheddar, 2% milk, sharp (Kraft), singles	1 slice	50	
Cheddar, 2% milk sharp (Kraft), shredded	¼ c	80	
Cheddar, mild (Organic Valley)	1 oz	110	
Cheddar, sharp (Organic Valley)	1 oz	110	
Cheddar, double, chef style (Sargento)	¼ c	110	
Cheddar, natural, mild, cubes (Sargento)	7 cubes	120	
Cheddar, sharp deli style, sliced (Sargento)	1 slice	80	
Colby (Organic Valley)	1 oz	110	
Colby, Longhorn, pre-sliced (Sara Lee)	1 slice	109	
Colby, deli style, sliced (Sargento)	1 slice	80	
Colby, natural Colby Jack cubes (Sargento)	7 cubes	110	
Cottage Cheese			
Breakstone's, small curd, f-f	5 oz	80	
Breakstone's, large curd, 2%	4 oz	90	
Breakstone's, small curd, 4%	4 oz	120	

Protein (g)	Total Fat (g)	Sat. Fat (g)	Trans Fat (g)	Chol. (mg)	Sodium (mg)	Calcium (%)	Iron (%)	Carbs (g)	Fiber (g)
6	6	4.5	0	20	300	15	na	1	0
4	2.5	1.5	0	10	300	25	na	2	0
3	4.5	2.5	0	15	250	20	na	1	0
4	7	4	0	20	340	10	na	0	0
12	9	6	0	30	430	20	na	0	0
4	6	3.5	0	20	240	15	na	<1	0
6	8	5	0	25	380	15	na	1	0
6	8	5	0	25	380	15	na	1	0
6	7	4	0	20	238	11	1	0	0
7	7	4.5	0	20	200	20	na	0	0
4	3	2	0	10	290	25	na	0	0
7	6	3.5	0	20	230	40	na	0	0
7	9	6	0	30	170	20	na	0	0
0	0	6	0	30	170	20	na	0	0
7	9	5	0	30	190	20	na	1	0
7	10	6	0	30	190	20	na	<1	0
5	6	4	0	20	140	15	na	0	0
7	9	6	0	20	230	40	na	0	0
7	9	5	0	30	170	na	na	0	0
5	7	4	0	20	140	15	na	0	0
6	9	6	0	25	200	20	na	0	0
12	0	0	0	10	450	15	0	8	0
11	2.5	1.5	0	15	410	15	0	6	0
12	5	3	0	25	430	15	0	6	0

Cheese

FOOD NAME	Portion Size	Calories
Breakstone's, Cottage Doubles, Blueberry	5.5 oz	140
Breakstone's, Cottage Doubles, Peach	5.5 oz	130
Breakstone's, Cottage Doubles, Strawberry	5.5 oz	130
Knudsen, free nonfat	½ c	80
Knudsen, small curd	½ c	120
Knudsen, small curd low fat (2%)	½ c	100
Knudsen, Cottage Doubles, Apples & Cinnamon	1 cont	140
Knudsen, Cottage Doubles, Blueberry	1 cont	140
Knudsen, Cottage Doubles, Peach	1 cont	140
Knudsen, Cottage Doubles, Pineapple	1 cont	130
Knudsen, Cottage Doubles, Raspberry	1 cont	150
Knudsen, Cottage Doubles, Strawberry	1 cont	140
Organic Valley, organic, small curd	½ c	100
Cream cheese (Philadelphia)		
Blueberry	1.2 oz	90
Fat Free	1 oz	30
Garden Vegetable	1.2 oz	90
Jalapeno Light	1.2 oz	60
Original	1 oz	100
Neufchatel ⅓ less fat	1 oz	70
Peaches 'n cream	1.2 oz	90
Salmon	1.2 oz	80
Whipped	¾ oz	60
Whipped, chives	¾ oz	60

Protein (g)	Total Fat (g)	Sat. Fat (g)	Trans Fat (g)	Chol. (mg)	Sodium (mg)	Calcium (%)	Iron (%)	Carbs (g)	Fiber (g)
11	2.5	1.5	0	15	400	15	0	18	0
11	2.5	1.5	0	15	400	15	0	16	0
11	2	1.5	0	15	400	15	0	17	0
13	0	0	0	5	430	15	0	7	0
13	5	3	0	25	430	15	0	5	0
14	2.5	1.5	0	15	440	15	0	6	0
11	2	1.5	0	15	400	15	0	18	0
11	2.5	1.5	0	15	400	15	0	18	1
11	2.5	1.5	0	15	390	8	0	17	0
11	2.5	1.5	0	15	390	8	0	17	0
11	2.5	1.5	0	15	400	8	2	20	0
11	2.5	1.5	0	15	400	8	2	19	0
15	2	1.5	0	10	450	8	0	4	0
1	7	4.5	0	30	110	2	0	5	0
4	0	0	0	5	200	15	0.	2	0
1	8	5	0	35	160	2	0	2	0
2	4.5	2.5	0	15	200	10	0	2	0
2	10	6	0	30	90	0	0	1	0
3	6	4	0	20	120	2	0	1	0
1	7	4	0	30	110	2	0	5	0
2	8	4.5	0	30	220	2	0	2	0
1	6	3.5	0	20	90	na	na	3	0
1	6	3.5	0	15	130	0	0	1	0

FOOD NAME	Portion Size	Calories	
Whipped, mixed berry	¾ oz	70	
Edam, specialty (Sara Lee)	1 oz	105	
Edam (Boar's Head)	1 oz	60	
Feta, mild (Athenos)	¼ c	91	
Feta (Boar's Head)	1 oz	60	
Feta Crumbles (Organic Valley)	1 oz	60	
Goat (Alta Dena)	1 oz	104	
Goat (Chavrie)	1.1 oz	50	
Gorgonzola Crumbles (Athenos)	1 oz	98	
Gouda (Boar's Head)	1 oz	110	
Gouda, specialty (Sara Lee)	1 oz	109	
Jarlsberg, deli style, sliced (Sargento)	1 oz	80	
Monterey Jack (Boar's Head)	1 oz	105	
Monterey Jack (Land-O-Lakes)	1 oz	110	
Monterey Jack, reduce fat, shredded (Organic Valley)	¼ c	80	
Mozzarella, singles, 2% (Kraft)	1 slice	50	
Mozzarella, string, part skim (Organic Valley)	1 oz	81	
Mozzarella, part skim, shredded (Organic Valley)	¼ c	60	
Mozzarella, fat-free, shredded (Polly-O)	1 oz	40	
Mozzarella, part skim (Polly-O)	1 oz	80	
Mozzarella, deli style, sliced (Sargento)	1 slice	60	
Muenster, reduced sodium (Alpine Lace)	1 slice	110	

Protein (g)	Total Fat (g)	Sat. Fat (g)	Trans Fat (g)	Chol. (mg)	Sodium (mg)	Calcium (%)	Iron (%)	Carbs (g)	Fiber (g)
3	5	3	0	15	55	0	0	3	0
8	8	5	0	25	284	na	na	0	0
5	4	2.5	0	10	360	na	na	0	0
6	7	4.5	0	20	220	na	na	1	0
5	4	2.5	0	10	360	na	na	1	0
5	4	2.5	0	10	430	10	na	<1	0
7	8	5	0	30	120	na	na	1	0
3	4	2.5	0	20	120	20	na	1	0
6	8	5	0	27	355	13	na	2	0
6	9	5	0	30	280	20	na	0	0
7	9	6	0	30	260	na	na	0	0
6	6	3.5	0	15	110	20	na	0	0
6	9	6	0	25	180	na	0	0	0
7	9	6	0	25	190	20	na	0	0
9	5	3.5	0	15	180	20	0	1	0
4	2.5	1.5	0	10	300	20	0	2	0
8	5	3	0	14	149	21	0	1	0
7	5	3	0	15	160	20	0	1	0
8	0	0	0	5	350	15	0	1	0
7	5	3.5	0	15	200	20	0	1	0
5	4	2.5	0	10	140	15	0	1	0
7	9	5	0	25	85	30	0	1	0

Cheese – Cheese Substitutes FOOD NAME	Portion Size	Calories	
Muenster (Boar's Head)	1 oz	100	
Muenster (Organic Valley)	1 oz	100	
Parmesan, shredded (Organic Valley)	¼ c	110	
Parmesan, grated (Polly-O)	5 g	20	
Parmesan & Romano, grated (Polly-O)	5 g	20	
Parmesan, grated (Sargento)	2 tsp	25	
Provolone, reduced fat and sodium (Alpine Lace)	1 slice	90	
Provolone (Organic Valley)	1 oz	102	
Ricotta, fat free (Polly-O)	¼ c	45	
Ricotta, part skim (Polly-O)	¼ c	90	
Ricotta, part skim (Sargento)	¼ c	70	
Ricotta, whole milk (Sargento)	¼ c	90	
Swiss, Baby Swiss (Boar's Head)	1 oz	110	
Swiss, singles 2% (Kraft)	1 slice	50	
Swiss, deli style (Sargento)	1 slice	110	
CHEESE SUBSTITUTES			
Almond Rella (Rella)	1 oz	102	
Better Than Cream Cheese, plain (Tofutti)			
Better Than Cream Cheese, French Onion (Tofutti)	2 Tbs	80	
Soy American (Tofutti)	1 slice	70	
Soy American (Smart Beat)	1 slice	25	
Soy Cheddar, Good Slice (Yves)	1 slice	36	
Soy Cheddar, Veggie Shreds (Galaxy)	1.1 oz	59	

Protein (g)	Total Fat (g)	Sat. Fat (g)	Trans Fat (g)	Chol. (mg)	Sodium (mg)	Calcium (%)	Iron (%)	Carbs (g)	Fiber (g)
6	8	5	0	25	180	20	0	0	0
7	8	5	0	25	180	20	0	0	0
10	7	4	0	20	350	35	0	0	0
2	1.5	1	0	5	85	6	0	0	0
2	1.5	1	0	5	85	na	na	0	0
2	1.5	1	0	5	80	6	0	0	0
7	6	3.5	0	15	180	20	0	1	0
7	8	5	0	20	250	20	0	<1	0
8	0	0	0	5	80	20	0	3	0
8	6	4	0	20	65	25	0	2	0
6	4.5	3	0	25	85	10	0	3	0
7	6	4	0	25	75	15	0	3	0
7	9	6	0	25	135	20	0	<1	0
4	2.5	1.5	0	10	310	25	0	2	0
7	9	6	0	25	135	20	0	<1	0
6	3.5	0	0	0	280	na	na	1	0
1	8	2	0	0	135	na	na	1	0
2	5	2	0	0	290	na	na	2	0
4	0	0	0	0	180	15	na	3	0
4	2	0	0	0	282	na	na	1	0
6	3	0	0	0	390	na	na	2	0

FOOD NAME	Portion Size	Calories
Cheese Substitutes – Cherries		
Soy Mozzarella, slices (Tofutti)	1 slice	70
Soy Parmesan, Mozzarella, Romano shreds (Galaxy)	1.1 oz	59
Soy Swiss, Good Slice (Yves)	1 slice	35
Tofu Rella (Rella)	1 oz	80
Vegan Rella (Rella)	1 oz	71
CHEESE SPREADS		
Alouette, Garlic & Herb	2 Tbs	70
Alouette, Spinach Florentine	2 Tbs	60
Alouette, Vegetable Garden	2 Tbs	60
Kraft, Bacon	2 Tbs	90
Kraft, Cheese Whiz, light	2 Tbs	80
Kraft, Cheese Whiz, original	2 Tbs	90
Kraft, Cheese Whiz, Salsa Con Queso	2 Tbs	90
Kraft, Pimento & Olive Spread	2 Tbs	80
Kraft, Roca Blue	2 Tbs	80
Kraft, Sharp Cheese Squeez-A-Snack	2 Tbs	90
Velveeta, light	2 Tbs	60
Velveeta, Mexican Mild	2 Tbs	90
Velveeta, original	2 Tbs	80
CHERRIES		
Raw, sour, red, pitted	1 c	77
Raw, sweet, red, pitted	1 c	91
Del Monte canned, dark sweet	½ c	100
Dole, frozen	1 c	90

Protein (g)	Total Fat (g)	Sat. Fat (g)	Trans Fat (g)	Chol. (mg)	Sodium (mg)	Calcium (%)	Iron (%)	Carbs (g)	Fiber (g)
2	5	3	0	0	290	na	na	2	0
6	3	0	0	0	390	na	na	2	0
4	2	0	0	0	262	na	na	2	0
6	5	1	0	0	280	na	na	3	0
1	3	0	0	0	220	na	na	10	0
1	7	4.5	0	30	135	2	na	1	0
1	6	3.5	0	25	85	2	na	1	0
1	6	4	0	30	130	2	na	1	0
5	8	5	0	25	570	na	na	1	0
6	3.5	2	0	20	500	15	0	6	0
3	7	4.5	0	30	490	10	0	4	0
4	7	4.5	0	na	440	na	na	0	0
2	6	4	0	20	170	na	na	3	0
3	7	4.5	0	20	340	na	na	3	0
5	8	5	0	na	440	na	na	0	0
5	3	2	0	15	420	na	na	4	0
5	6	4	0	25	420	na	na	3	0
5	6	4	0	15	420	na	na	3	0
2	0	0	0	0	5	2	3	19	2
2	0	0	0	0	0	2	3	23	3
<1	0	0	0	0	10	0	2	24	<1
2	0	0	0	0	0	0	2	22	3

FOOD NAME	Portion Size	Calories	
S&W, dark & sweet	½ c	140	
CHERRY BEVERAGES			
Hi-C Wild Cherry, drink box	200 mL	100	
Knudsen, Black Cherry Spritzer	12 oz	180	
Knudsen, Cherry Cider	8 oz	130	
Knudsen, Just Black Cherry	8 oz	180	
Knudsen, Just Tart Cherry, organic	8 oz	130	
Kool-Aid	8 oz	80	
Minute Maid Cooler, Clear Cherry, pouch	200 ml	100	
CHESTNUTS			
Chinese, roasted	1 oz	68	
European, roasted	1 oz	69	
Japanese, roasted	1 oz	57	
CHICKEN, canned, Swanson			
Chicken a la King	10.5 oz	210	
Swanson Chicken Breast in Water	2 oz	50	
CHICKEN, fresh, boiler or fryer			
Breast & skin, roasted	4 oz	224	
Breast only, roasted	4 oz	188	
Dark & skin, roasted	4 oz	284	
Dark only, roasted	4 oz	232	
Drumstick, no skin, fried	1 pc	82	
Leg, no skin, fried	1 pc	196	
Light meat, no skin, fried	1 c	269	
Thigh, no skin, fried	1 pc	113	

Protein (g)	Total Fat (g)	Sat. Fat (g)	Trans Fat (g)	Chol. (mg)	Sodium (mg)	Calcium (%)	Iron (%)	Carbs (g)	Fiber (g)
1	0	0	0	0	10	0	2	34	1
0	0	0	0	0	0	0	0	15	0
<1	0	0	0	0	30	4	4	46	0
<1	0	0	0	0	40	2	4	33	0
2	0	0	0	0	40	2	0	44	0
1	0	0	0	0	20	2	8	32	0
0	0	0	0	0	0	0	0	20	0
0	0	0	0	0	0	10	0	15	0
1	0	0	0	0	1	1	2	15	0
1	0	0	0	0	1	1	1	15	1
1	0	0	0	0	5	1	3	13	0
14	12	3.5	0	20	1370	0	0	12	2
10	1	0.5	0	20	270	0	0	1	0
32	8	4	0	96	80	0	8	0	0
36	4	0	0	96	84	0	8	0	0
28	16	4	0	104	100	0	8	0	0
32	12	4	0	104	104	0	8	0	0
12	3	1	0	39	40	1	3	0	0
27	9	2	0	93	90	1	7	1	0
46	8	2	0	126	113	2	9	1	0
15	5	1	0	53	4	1	4	1	0

FOOD NAME	Portion Size	Calories	
CHICKEN, other			
Capon, meat & skin, roasted	4 oz	260	
Cornish Game Hen, roasted	1 bird	295	
Giblets, simmered	1 c	281	
Liver, simmered	4 oz	188	
CHICKEN, refrigerated or frozen			
Organic Valley, ground, frozen	4 oz	200	
Organic Valley, breast, boneless, skinless	4 oz	120	
Perdue, breast nuggets, cooked	5 pc	248	
Perdue, breast tenderloins, skinless, boneless	3 oz	101	
Perdue, Cornish Hens, cooked	3 oz	210	
Tyson			
Breast fillet	1 pc	240	
Breast fillet, Mesquite	1 pc	130	
Breast, diced strips	3 oz	68	
Chicken Bites	3 oz	270	
Nuggets, frozen	5 pcs	280	
Strips, Buffalo Style	2 pcs	230	
Strips, Crispy Chicken	2 pcs	200	
Tenders, Honey Battered	5 pcs	220	
Wings, Hot 'n Spicy	3 pcs	219	
Weaver			
Breast Strips	3 pcs	230	
Breast Tenders	5 pcs	240	

Protein (g)	Total Fat (g)	Sat. Fat (g)	Trans Fat (g)	Chol. (mg)	Sodium (mg)	Calcium (%)	Iron (%)	Carbs (g)	Fiber (g)
32	12	4	0	96	56	0	8	0	0
51	9	2	0	233	139	3	9	0	0
37	13	4	0	515	81	2	52	0	0
28	8	4	0	636	84	0	72	0	0
21	12	3	0	95	90	20	na	1	0
26	1.5	0	0	65	75	na	na	0	0
11	16	3.5	0	40	720	0	na	15	1
23	1	0.5	0	55	100	0	na	0	0
21	14	4.5	0	125	55	0	na	0	0
19	09	1.5	0	30	680	0	na	20	0
17	7	2	0	45	540	0	na	1	0
20	15	3.5	0	34	188	0	na	0	0
13	18	4	0	40	400	6	6	12	1
14	18	4	0	40	400	0	na	16	0
14	10	2	0	40	1250	0	na	21	14
16	10	2	0	30	520	0	na	13	1
13	13	3	0	35	250	0	na	13	2
20	15	3.5	0	110	560	0	na	1	0
12	14	3.5	0	35	620	na	na	14	1
12	14	3	0	35	330	na	na	15	0

Chicken, refrigerated or frozen – Chili & Chili Beans FOOD NAME	Portion Size	Calories	
Buffalo Popcorn Chicken	7 pcs	230	
Crispy Mini-Drums	5 pcs	250	
Italian Style Patties	1	210	
Nuggets	4 pcs	210	
Original Patties	1	180	
CHICKEN SUBSTITUTES			
Morningstar			
Buffalo wings	5 wings	200	
Chik 'n Nuggets	4 pcs	190	
Chik 'n Patties	1	160	
Chik 'n Tenders	2 pcs	190	
Worthington			
Chik Sticks	6 pcs	100	
Diced Chik, fat free	¼ c	30	
Fried Chik 'n Gravy	2 pcs	150	
Meatless Chicken Roll	⅜" slice	90	
Meatless Chicken Slices	3 slices	90	
CHICKPEAS (Garbanzo Beans)			
Eden, organic	½ c	130	
Progresso	½ c	100	
S&W	½ c	80	
CHILIS, green, canned			
Pace, diced	2 Tbs	10	
Old El Paso, whole	1	10	
CHILI & CHILI BEANS			

Protein (g)	Total Fat (g)	Sat. Fat (g)	Trans Fat (g)	Chol. (mg)	Sodium (mg)	Calcium (%)	Iron (%)	Carbs (g)	Fiber (g)
14	14	2	0	35	900	0	0	13	1
14	16	3.5	0	40	410	2	4	14	1
10	14	3	0	20	470	6	6	12	1
11	15	3.5	0	35	360	na	na	9	1
10	11	2.5	0	30	430	2	6	10	1
12	9	1.5	0	0	630	2	15	18	3
12	7	1	0	0	400	2	15	18	2
11	6	1	0	0	430	4	10	15	2
12	7	1	0	0	580	4	10	20	3
10	6	1	0	0	300	2	10	4	2
9	0	0	0	0	220	0	6	2	1
12	10	1.5	0	0	430	2	10	5	2
9	4.5	0.5	0	0	240	10	6	2	1
9	4.5	1	0	0	250	25	10	2	<1
7	1	0	0	0	30	6	8	23	5
5	1.5	0	0	0	280	2	6	17	4
7	1	0	0	0	46	02	6	19	5
0	0	0	0	0	100	0	0	2	<1
0	0	0	0	0	230	0	0	2	0

FOOD NAME	Portion Size	Calories	
Eden Organic Chili Beans w/ Jalapeno & Red Pepper	½ c	130	
Campbell's Chunky, Firehouse	1 c	220	
Campbell's Chunky, Roadhouse	1 c	220	
Campbell's Sizzling Steak	1 c	200	
Fantastic Foods, Vegetarian Chili	1 c	200	
Health Valley, 99% f-f Vegetarian Spicy Black Bean	1 c	160	
Health Valley, 99% f-f Medium Turkey Chili	1 c	220	
Health Valley, Mild Vegetarian Chili	1 c	160	
Health Valley, Vegetarian Lentil Chili	1 c	160	
S&W, Chili Beans, Santa Fe	½ c	90	
S&W, Chili Beans, Tomato Sauce	½ c	110	
Stagg, Classic Chili	1 c	330	
Stagg, Country Brand	1 c	320	
Stagg, Laredo	1 c	320	
Stagg, Ranch House Chicken Chili	1 c	290	
Stagg, Turkey Ranchero	1 c	240	
Stagg, Vegetable Garden 4-Bean	1 c	200	
CHOCOLATE, baking			
Baker's Baking Unsweetened Squares	½ oz	70	
Baker's Bittersweet Squares	½ oz	70	
Baker's Chocolate Chunks Semi-Sweet	½ oz	70	
Baker's German's Sweet	½ oz	60	
Baker's Premium White Squares	½ oz	80	

Protein (g)	Total Fat (g)	Sat. Fat (g)	Trans Fat (g)	Chol. (mg)	Sodium (mg)	Calcium (%)	Iron (%)	Carbs (g)	Fiber (g)
9	0	0	0	0	250	6	15	21	7
15	8	3.5	0	25	750	4	10	21	8
15	8	3.5	0	25	750	4	10	21	8
13	3.5	1.5	0	15	880	4	10	28	6
16	2	0	0	0	1160	10	25	32	7
13	1	0	0	0	320	4	20	28	12
16	3	1	0	0	480	8	25	34	8
14	1	0	0	0	390	4	30	30	11
15	1	0	0	0	390	4	20	28	11
7	0	0	0	0	570	8	10	21	6
7	1	0	0	0	580	4	8	23	6
17	17	8	0	45	820	6	15	28	5
15	16	7	0	45	1130	4	15	20	5
18	15	7	0	45	1150	4	10	27	6
19	9	3	0	50	810	6	15	32	6
22	3	1	0	35	880	6	10	31	6
10	1	0	0	0	870	6	15	37	7
2	7	4.5	0	0	0	0	8	4	2
1	6	3	0	0	0	na	2	7	1
1	4.5	2.5	0	0	5	0	4	0	0
1	3.5	2	0	0	0	0	2	8	1
1	4.5	3	0	5	15	2	0	8	0

FOOD NAME	Portion Size	Calories	
CLAMS			
Bumble Bee, canned	¼ c	50	
Chicken of the Sea, chopped	¼ c	30	
Chicken of the Sea, Whole Baby	¼ c	30	
Mrs. Paul's Fried Clams	3 oz	270	
COCONUT			
Fresh, raw, shredded	1 c	283	
Baker's Angel Flake, shredded, sweetened	2 oz	70	
Milk, Organic Lite (Thai Kitchen)	2 oz	45	
COD			
Atlantic, baked	3 oz	89	
Atlantic, canned	3 oz	89	
Pacific, baked	3 oz	89	
COFFEE, flavored, General Foods			
International			
Café Francais	1 serv	60	
Crème Caramel	1 serv	60	
French Vanilla	1 serv	60	
French Vanilla, sugar free	1 serv	30	
French Vanilla Nut	1 serv	60	
Italian Cappuccino	1 serv	50	
Suisse Mocha	1 serv	60	
Viennese Chocolate	1 serv	50	
COLLARDS, fresh, cooked, no salt	1 c	49	
COOKIES, mixes and unbaked			

Protein (g)	Total Fat (g)	Sat. Fat (g)	Trans Fat (g)	Chol. (mg)	Sodium (mg)	Calcium (%)	Iron (%)	Carbs (g)	Fiber (g)
9	1	0.5	0	40	270	6	90	2	0
5	0	0	0	12	370	0	2	2	0
6	0	0	0	10	290	0	6	1	0
9	13	2.5	0	20	690	0	10	20	1
3	27	24	0	0	16	1	11	12	7
1	5	4.5	0	0	40	0	0	6	1
0	3	3	0	0	12	15	na	1	0
19	1	0	0	47	66	1	2	0	0
19	1	0	0	47	185	2	2	0	0
20	1	0	0	40	77	1	2	0	0
0	3	2.5	0	na	90	na	na	8	na
0	2	1.5	0	0	50	na	na	12	na
0	2.5	0.5	0	na	55	na	na	10	na
0	2.5	2	0	0	50	na	na	2	na
0	2.5	2.5	0	0	55	na	na	10	na
0	1.5	1.5	0	0	45	na	na	10	na
0	2	1.5	0	0	40	na	na	10	na
0	1.5	1.5	0	0	25	na	na	11	na
4	1	0	0	0	30	27	12	9	5

Cookies, mixes and unbaked – Cookies, ready-to-eat

FOOD NAME	Portion Size	Calories	
Betty Crocker			
Chocolate Chip, pouch	2	120	
Chocolate Peanut Butter Chip, pouch	2	120	
Oatmeal, pouch	2	110	
Peanut Butter, pouch	2	120	
Sugar, pouch	2	120	
Pillsbury			
Big Deluxe Classic, Chocolate	1	200	
Big Deluxe Classic, Peanut Butter Cup	1	190	
Big Deluxe Classic, Turtle Supreme	1	200	
Chocolate Chip, bake	1 oz	130	
Chocolate Chip Walnut	1	120	
Oatmeal Chocolate Chip	1 oz	130	
Ready to Bake Chocolate Candy	1	120	
Ready to Bake Chocolate Chunk & Chip	1	120	
Ready to Bake, Sugar	1	120	
COOKIES, ready-to-eat			
Archway, Double Fudge Crème	2	190	
Archway, Fig Bars	2	110	
Barbara's			
Animal Cookies	8	120	
Chocolate Chip	1	80	
Fig bar, Apple Cinnamon	1	60	
Fig Bar, Blueberry	1	70	
Fig Bar, Raspberry	1	60	

Protein (g)	Total Fat (g)	Sat. Fat (g)	Trans Fat (g)	Chol. (mg)	Sodium (mg)	Calcium (%)	Iron (%)	Carbs (g)	Fiber (g)
1	3	1.5	0	0	100	na	6	21	na
2	3.5	2.5	0	0	110	na	4	20	<1
2	1.5	0	0	0	100	na	2	22	<1
2	4	1	0	0	140	na	2	20	na
1	2.5	0.5	0	0	65	na	2	20	na
2	10	3.5	2	10	130	0	4	25	1
3	9	3.5	1.5	5	160	0	4	24	<1
2	10	3.5	1.5	5	120	2	4	25	<1
1	7	2	1.5	5	85	0	4	17	<1
1	7	2	1	<5	80	0	2	14	<1
1	6	2	1	5	95	0	2	17	<1
1	5	2	1	5	70	0	2	16	0
1	6	2	1.5	<5	80	0	4	15	0
1	6	1.5	1.5	5	70	0	2	15	0
2	9	4	1.5	0	120	0	6	26	1
1	2	0	0	0	85	2	4	23	1
2	4.5	2.5	0	10	85	2	0	18	<1
1	4	2	0	0	40	0	2	9	<1
1	0	0	0	0	25	0	2	14	1
0	0.5	0	0	0	20	0	2	15	0
1	0	0	0	0	25	0	2	14	1

Cookies, ready-to-eat FOOD NAME	Portion Size	Calories	
Fig bar, Traditional	1	60	
Fig Bar, Wheat Free	1	60	
Fig Bar, Whole Wheat	1	60	
Double Dutch Chocolate	1	80	
Old-Fashioned Oatmeal	1	70	
Snackimals, Chocolate Chip	10	120	
Snackimals, Vanilla	10	110	
Snackimals, Wheat-Free	10	120	
Traditional Shortbread	1	80	
Famous Amos			
Chocolate Chip & Pecans	4	150	
Chocolate Crème Sandwich	3	160	
Iced Gingersnaps, low-fat	2 oz	200	
Oatmeal Chocolate Chip Walnut	4	140	
Oatmeal Raisin	4	140	
Vanilla Crème Sandwich	3	170	
Health Valley			
Apricot Delight, f-f	3	100	
Café Creations Chocolate Chip	1	100	
Chocolate Chip Oatmeal	1	100	
Chocolate Vanilla Cream Cookie Bar	1	200	
Cookie Crème Chocolate Sandwich	2	120	
Oatmeal Raisin	1	90	
White Chocolate Chunk	1	140	
Keebler			

Protein (g)	Total Fat (g)	Sat. Fat (g)	Trans Fat (g)	Chol. (mg)	Sodium (mg)	Calcium (%)	Iron (%)	Carbs (g)	Fiber (g)
0	0.5	0	0	0	20	0	2	14	0
1	0	0	0	0	25	0	2	13	1
1	0	0	0	0	25	0	4	13	1
1	4	2.5	0	10	45	0	3	9	<1
<1	3	1.5	0	5	75	0	1	11	<1
1	4	0	0	0	80	0	4	19	0
2	4	0	0	0	65	4	8	17	0
1	5	0	0	0	130	4	8	17	1
1	4	3	0	10	45	0	0	9	<1
2	8	2.5	1.5	0	105	0	2	18	<1
2	6	1.5	2.5	0	140	0	6	25	<1
3	3	0.5	1	0	170	0	6	40	1
2	6	2	2	<5	130	0	2	18	1
2	6	2	2	<5	130	0	2	20	<1
1	7	1.5	2.5	0	85	0	2	25	0
2	0	0	0	0	90	na	4	24	3
1	5	2	0	5	50	2	6	13	2
2	4	0.5	0	0	50	15	6	14	1
2	8	2.5	0	20	90	2	15	32	1
1	4	1	0	0	100	na	8	19	0
2	3.5	0	0	0	50	15	4	14	1
1	7	3	0	10	150	na	6	17	0

Cookies, ready-to-eat FOOD NAME	Portion Size	Calories	
Animal Cookies, Frosted	8	150	
Chip Deluxe, Chocolate Lovers	1	80	
Chips Deluxe Coconut	1	80	
Chips Deluxe, Peanut Butter Cups	1	90	
E.L. Fudge Double Stuffed	2	180	
Fudge Shoppe, Deluxe Graham	3	140	
Fudge Shoppe, Filled Peanut Butter	2	170	
Fudge Shoppe, Fudge Sticks	3	150	
Fudge Shoppe, reduced fat, Fudge Stripes	3	130	
Golden Vanilla Wafers	8	140	
Oatmeal, Country Style	2	130	
Sandies, Chocolate Chip Pecan	1	80	
Sandies, Fruit Delights, Strawberry Cheesecake	1	80	
Sandies, Pecan	1	80	
Sandies, Pecan, reduced fat	1	80	
Sandies, Simply Shortbread	1	80	
Sandies, Swirl Cinnamon	1	90	
Soft Batch, Chocolate Chip	1	80	
Soft Batch, Oatmeal Raisin	1	80	
Vienna Fingers	2	150	
Vienna Fingers, reduced fat	2	140	
Murray Sugar Free			
Chocolate Chip	3	140	
Chocolate Sandwich Cream	3	130	

Protein (g)	Total Fat (g)	Sat. Fat (g)	Trans Fat (g)	Chol. (mg)	Sodium (mg)	Calcium (%)	Iron (%)	Carbs (g)	Fiber (g)
1	7	4.5	1.5	0	80	0	2	22	<1
1	4.5	2	1	<5	65	0	2	10	<1
1	4.5	2	1.5	0	50	0	2	10	<1
1	4.5	2	1.5	0	50	0	2	10	<1
2	9	2	3.5	<5	90	0	2	23	<5
1	7	4.5	1.5	0	70	0	2	17	<1
3	11	5	0.5	0	100	0	2	15	<1
<1	8	4.5	2	0	30	0	2	19	0
1	5	3	1	0	105	0	4	21	<1
1	6	1	2.5	0	120	0	2	21	<1
2	6	1.5	2.5	0	115	0	4	18	1
<1	5	1	1.5	0	50	0	2	9	0
0	3.5	1	1	<5	55	0	0	11	0
<1	5	1	2	<5	50	0	0	9	0
<1	3.5	0.5	1.5	0	65	0	2	11	0
<1	4.5	2	1	5	65	0	2	10	0
<1	5	1	2	<5	55	0	2	10	<1
<1	3.5	1	1	0	55	0	2	11	<1
1	3	0.5	1	0	65	0	0	11	<1
1	7	1.5	2.5	0	95	0	2	22	<1
1	5	1	2	0	115	0	2	24	<1
2	7	2	2	0	85	0	4	23	2
1	7	1.5	2.5	0	85	0	4	18	1

Cookies, ready-to-eat	Portion Size	Calories	
Double Fudge	3	140	
Lemon Wafers	4	130	
Oatmeal	3	150	
Peanut Butter	3	140	
Shortbread	8	140	
Shortbread Pecan	3	170	
Vanilla Wafers	9	130	
Nabisco			
Chips Ahoy, 100% whole grain	1	150	
Chips Ahoy, Chocolate Chip	2	160	
Chips Ahoy, Chunky Chocolate Chip	1	80	
Chips Ahoy, Chunky White Fudge	1	80	
Chips Ahoy, reduced fat	1	140	
Chips Ahoy, Soft Baked Chunky	1	120	
Fig Newtons, 100% whole grain	2	110	
Fig Newtons, f-f	2	90	
Fig Newtons, original	2	110	
Nilla Wafers, original	1 oz	140	
Nilla Wafers, reduced fat	1 oz	120	
Nutter Butter sandwich	2	130	
Oreo Sandwich	3	160	
Oreo Sandwich, Chocolate Crème	2	110	
Oreo Sandwich, Double Stuf	2	140	
Oreo Sandwich, reduced fat	3	150	
Snackwell's, Crème Sandwich	2	110	

Protein (g)	Total Fat (g)	Sat. Fat (g)	Trans Fat (g)	Chol. (mg)	Sodium (mg)	Calcium (%)	Iron (%)	Carbs (g)	Fiber (g)
2	7	2	2	0	85	0	4	23	2
1	8	1.5	3	0	20	0	2	20	5
2	8	1.5	2.5	0	160	0	4	21	2
3	0	?	2	<5	135	0	2	16	1
2	6	1.5	2	0	140	0	4	21	1
2	11	2.5	3.5	<5	110	0	4	18	1
2	5	1.5	2	<5	80	0	4	24	1
2	8	2.5	0	0	110	0	4	22	2
2	8	2.5	0	0	110	0	4	22	1
1	4	1.5	0	0	55	0	2	10	1
1	4.5	1.5	0	0	60	0	2	11	0
2	5	2	0	0	150	0	4	23	1
1	5	2.5	0	0	100	2	4	19	1
1	2	0.5	0	0	115	2	4	21	0
1	0	0	0	0	125	4	4	22	1
1	2	0	0	0	120	2	4	22	1
1	6	1.5	0	5	115	2	4	21	0
1	2	0	0	0	110	0	4	24	0
2	5	1.5	0	0	110	0	4	19	<1
2	7	2	0	0	180	0	10	25	1
1	3	0.5	0	0	130	0	2	20	0
1	7	2.5	0	0	130	0	6	20	<1
2	4.5	1	0	0	190	0	10	26	1
1	3	0.5	0	0	130	0	2	20	0

FOOD NAME	Portion Size	Calories	
Snackwell's, Devil's Food, f-f	1	50	
Pepperidge Farm			
Bordeaux	4	130	
Brussels	3	150	
Chocolate Chunk Milk Chocolate			
Macadamia	1	140	
Chocolate Chunk White Chocolate			
Macadamia	1	130	
Double Chocolate Chunk, Dark Chocolate	1	140	
Geneva	3	160	
Gingerbread Man	4	130	
Milano Double Chocolate	2	140	
Milano, original	3	180	
Shortbread	2	140	
Soft Bake, Chocolate Chunk	1	150	
Soft Bake, Snickerdoodle	1	140	
Soft Bake, Sugar	1	140	
Sugar	3	140	
Verona Strawberry	3	140	
CORN			
Fresh, cooked, white or yellow, no salt	1 c	177	
Fresh, cooked, white or yellow	7" cob	111	
Canned			
Del Monte, Savory Sides, in Butter Sauce	½ c	90	
Del Monte, Savory Sides, Fiesta Corn	½ c	50	

Protein (g)	Total Fat (g)	Sat. Fat (g)	Trans Fat (g)	Chol. (mg)	Sodium (mg)	Calcium (%)	Iron (%)	Carbs (g)	Fiber (g)
1	0	0	0	0	30	0	2	12	0
2	5	3.5	0	10	95	0	2	19	<1
2	7	4	0	5	65	0	4	20	1
2	8	3.5	0	10	80	0	4	16	0
1	6	4	0	<5	85	0	6	17	<1
2	7	3	0	10	80	0	6	18	1
2	9	4	0	0	95	0	6	19	1
2	4	2	0	10	100	0	4	21	<1
2	8	4	0	10	70	0	4	17	<1
2	10	5	0	10	80	0	6	21	<1
2	7	4	0	10	105	0	2	16	<1
2	8	3.5	0	10	95	0	4	22	<1
2	5	2.5	0	10	95	0	4	22	<1
2	5	2.5	0	10	90	0	4	22	0
2	6	2.5	0	15	90	0	4	20	<1
2	5	2.5	0	10	100	0	2	22	<1
5	2	0	0	0	28	0	6	41	4
3	1	0	0	0	18	0	3	26	3
2	2.5	1	0	5	530	0	2	14	<1
2	1	0	0	0	310	0	2	12	2

Corn

FOOD NAME	Portion Size	Calories
Del Monte, Savory Sides, gold & white	½ c	80
Del Monte, Savory Sides, Santa Fe	½ c	70
Del Monte, Savory Sides, white, cream	½ c	100
Del Monte, Savory Sides, whole kernel	½ c	90
Green Giant, Créamed Corn	½ c	90
Green Giant, Extra Sweet Niblets	⅓ c	50
Green Giant, Mexicorn	⅓ c	70
Green Giant, Whole Kernel Sweet	½ c	80
S&W, Creamed Corn	½ c	60
S&W, Whole Kernels	½ c	80
Frozen		
Birds Eye, Baby Gold & White	⅔ c	100
Birds Eye, Baby White Corn Kernels	⅔ c	90
Birds Eye, Baby Corn & Vegetable Blend	¾ c	70
Birds Eye, Super Sweet Kernel Corn	⅔ c	70
Birds Eye, Sweet Corn & Bacon in Cheese Sauce	½ c	150
Birds Eye, Sweet Corn & Butter Sauce	½ c	150
Birds Eye, Sweet Kernel Corn	⅔ c	100
Cascadian Farms, Organic Sweet Corn	¾ c	70
C&W, Salsa Corn	1 c	90
Green Giant, Cob, Niblets	1 ear	150
Green Giant, Cream Style	½ c	110
Green Giant, Niblets w/ Butter	⅔ c	110
Green Giant, Shoepeg White Corn, no sauce	½ c	70

Protein (g)	Total Fat (g)	Sat. Fat (g)	Trans Fat (g)	Chol. (mg)	Sodium (mg)	Calcium (%)	Iron (%)	Carbs (g)	Fiber (g)
2	0.5	0	0	0	360	0	2	18	2
3	1	0	0	0	510	0	4	16	1
2	1	0	0	0	360	0	2	21	2
2	1	0	0	0	360	0	2	18	3
2	0.5	0	0	0	400	0	0	19	1
2	0.5	0	0	0	200	0	0	10	1
2	0.5	0	0	0	250	0	0	14	1
2	0.5	0	0	0	360	0	0	18	2
1	0.5	0	0	0	360	0	2	14	2
2	1	0	0	0	360	0	2	11	3
3	1	0	0	0	0	0	2	20	2
3	1	0	0	0	0	0	2	18	3
2	0	0	0	0	0	2	2	13	2
3	1	0	0	0	0	0	2	14	2
5	4	1.5	0	5	470	4	2	26	1
3	3	1	0	0	260	0	0	28	2
3	1	0	0	0	0	0	0	21	1
3	0.5	0	0	0	0	0	2	18	2
3	0.5	0	0	0	250	2	4	17	3
4	1	0	0	0	10	4	10	32	3
2	1	0	0	0	330	0	0	23	2
3	1.5	0.5	0	<5	340	0	0	22	2
2	1	0	0	0	45	0	0	15	2

FOOD NAME	Portion Size	Calories	
CORN CHIPS			
Bugles, Chili Cheese	1⅓ c	160	
Bugles, Original	1⅓ c	160	
Bugles, Salsa	1⅓ c	160	
Bugles, Smokin' BBQ	1⅓ c	150	
Bugles, Southwest Ranch	1⅓ c	170	
Doritos, Cool Ranch Tortilla	1 oz	140	
Doritos, Cool Ranch Tortilla, baked	1 oz	120	
Doritos, Light Nacho Cheese	1 oz	100	
Doritos, Nacho Cheese Tortilla	1 oz	140	
Doritos, Nacho Cheese Tortilla, baked	1 oz	120	
Doritos, Ranchero Tortilla	1 oz	150	
Doritos, Rollitos Cooler Ranch	1 oz	150	
Doritos, Rollitos Nacho Cheesier	1 oz	150	
Doritos, Rollitos, Zesty Taco	1 oz	150	
Doritos, Spicy Nacho	1 oz	140	
Doritos, Toasted Corn	1 oz	140	
Fritos, Bar-B-Q	1 oz	150	
Fritos, Cheese Flavor	1 oz	160	
Fritos, Flamin' Hot	1 oz	160	
Fritos, King Size	1 oz	160	
Fritos, Original	1 oz	160	
Fritos, Scoops	1 oz	160	
Herr's, Bite Size Dippers	1 oz	140	
Herr's, Corn Chips	1 oz	160	

Protein (g)	Total Fat (g)	Sat. Fat (g)	Trans Fat (g)	Chol. (mg)	Sodium (mg)	Calcium (%)	Iron (%)	Carbs (g)	Fiber (g)
2	9	7	0	0	310	na	na	18	na
1	9	8	0	0	310	na	N	18	<1
2	9	7	0	0	320	na	na	18	na
1	8	7	0	0	360	na	na	18	na
1	10	8	0	0	310	na	na	18	na
2	7	1	0	0	170	2	2	18	1
2	3.5	−.5	0	0	200	4	4	21	2
2	2	0.5	0	0	200	2	2	19	2
2	8	1.5	0	0	180	2	2	17	1
2	3.5	0.5	0	0	220	4	4	21	2
2	8	1	0	0	290	0	2	17	1
2	8	1.5	0	0	140	2	2	17	1
2	8	1.5	0	0	200	0	2	17	1
2	8	1.5	0	0	140	2	2	17	1
2	7	1	0	0	210	4	2	18	<1
2	7	1	0	0	120	4	0	18	1
2	10	1.5	0	0	280	4	2	16	1
2	10	1.5	0	0	260	4	0	15	1
2	10	1.5	0	0	160	4	0	15	1
2	10	1.5	0	0	150	2	0	16	1
2	10	1.5	0	0	170	2	0	15	1
2	10	1.5	0	0	110	4	0	16	1
3	6	1.5	0	0	90	4	2	18	2
2	10	2	0	0	170	4	4	17	2

FOOD NAME	Portion Size	Calories	
Herr's, Mexican Cheddar Dippers	1 oz	150	
Herr's, Nachitos	1 oz	140	
Tostitos, Natural Blue Corn	1 oz	140	
Tostitos, Original Bite Size, baked	1 oz	110	
Tostitos, Restaurant Style Tortilla	1 oz	140	
Tostitos, Santa Fe Rounds	1 oz	140	
Tostitos, Sensations Red Chile & Lime	1 oz	150	
Tostitos, Sensations Southwestern Ranch	1 oz	150	
Wise, Dipsy Doodles, rippled	1 oz	160	
Wise, Nacho Twister	1 oz	160	
COUSCOUS			
Fantastic Foods			
Organic, prep	¼ c	150	
Organic, whole wheat, uncooked	¼ c	170	
Near East			
Herb Chicken, mix	2 oz	190	
Mediterranean Curry, mix	2 oz	190	
Original Plain, dry	⅓ c	220	
Parmesan, mix	2 oz	200	
Toasted Pine Nut, mix	2 oz	200	
Tomato Lentil, mix	2 oz	190	
CRAB			
Bumble Bee, canned, white	¼ c	40	
Chicken of the Sea, canned, fancy	2 oz	40	
Fresh, cooked, blue	1 c	120	

Protein (g)	Total Fat (g)	Sat. Fat (g)	Trans Fat (g)	Chol. (mg)	Sodium (mg)	Calcium (%)	Iron (%)	Carbs (g)	Fiber (g)
2	7	2	0	0	230	4	2	18	2
2	6	1	0	0	230	4	2	18	2
2	6	0.5	0	0	80	2	2	19	1
3	1	0	0	0	200	4	2	24	2
2	7	1	0	0	120	4	2	19	1
1	6	1	0	0	80	2	0	20	1
2	8	1	0	0	65	2	2	17	2
2	8	1.5	0	0	130	2	2	18	2
1	10	2.5	0	0	180	2	2	16	1
1	11	3	0	0	250	4	2	14	1
0	0.5	0	0	0	0	0	4	33	1
7	0.5	0	0	0	0	2	8	37	6
8	1	0	0	0	510	2	6	40	3
8	1	0	0	0	550	2	8	40	3
8	1	0	0	0	5	0	6	46	2
8	2	0	0	0	510	2	6	39	2
8	3	0.5	0	0	510	2	6	38	3
8	1	0	0	0	670	2	6	40	3
8	1	0	0	50	300	2	2	0	0
7	0	0	0	50	400	6	2	2	0
24	2	0	0	118	329	12	6	0	0

Crab – Crackers FOOD NAME	Portion Size	Calories	
Fresh, cooked, Dungeness	3 oz	93	
CRACKERS			
Eden Foods, Brown Rice	8	120	
Eden Foods, Nori Maki Rice	15	110	
Health Valley			
Bruschetta Vegetable, no salt added	6	60	
Butter Corn Bread Crackers	4	60	
Garden Herb, low-fat	5	60	
Honey Corn Bread Crackers	4	60	
Original Oat Bran Graham	6	120	
Sesame, low-fat	5	60	
Stoned Wheat, low-fat	5	60	
Keebler			
Club, original	4	70	
Club, reduced fat	5	70	
Grahams, Cinnamon Crisp, low-fat	8	110	
Grahams, Honey	8	140	
Grahams, original	8	130	
Scooby-Doo Graham Cracker Sticks	9	130	
Scooby-Doo Graham Cracker			
Sticks, honey	9	130	
Sunshine, Cheez-It, Cheddar Jack	25	160	
Sunshine, Cheez-It, Fiesta Cheddar Nacho	25	160	
Sunshine, Cheez-It, Hot & Spicy	25	150	
Sunshine, Cheez-It, original	27	160	

Protein (g)	Total Fat (g)	Sat. Fat (g)	Trans Fat (g)	Chol. (mg)	Sodium (mg)	Calcium (%)	Iron (%)	Carbs (g)	Fiber (g)
19	1	0	0	65	321	5	2	1	0
3	2	0	0	0	230	2	4	2	2
3	0	0	0	0	160	4	2	24	2
2	1.5	0	0	0	40	2	2	10	1
1	1.5	0	0	0	160	2	2	11	1
2	1.5	0	0	0	140	2	2	10	1
1	1.5	0	0	0	140	2	2	11	1
3	3	0	0	0	80	4	4	22	3
2	1.5	0	0	0	140	2	2	10	1
1	1	0	0	0	140	2	2	10	1
1	3	1	0	0	150	0	2	9	<1
1	2.5	0.5	0	0	190	0	2	12	<1
2	1.5	0	0	0	140	10	4	23	1
2	4	1	0	0	150	10	6	23	<1
2	3.5	1	0	0	160	10	6	22	<1
2	4	0.5	0	0	120	10	4	21	<1
2	4	0.5	0	0	120	10	4	21	<1
3	8	2.5	0	0	250	4	4	18	0
3	8	2.5	0	0	280	0	6	20	<1
2	8	2	0	0	280	0	8	18	<1
4	8	2	0	0	250	4	4	18	<1

Crackers / FOOD NAME	Portion Size	Calories	
Sunshine, Cheez-It, reduced fat	29	130	
Sunshine, Cheez-It, Twisterz Cool Ranch	17	140	
Sunshine, Cheez-It, Twisterz, Hot Wings			
Cheesy Blue	17	140	
Sunshine, Cheez-It, White Cheddar	25	150	
Sunshine, Krispy, original	5	60	
Sunshine, Krispy, Soup & Oyster	5	70	
Sunshine, Krispy, Whole Wheat	5	60	
Toasteds, Buttercrisp	5	80	
Toasteds, Onion	5	80	
Toasteds, Sesame	5	80	
Toasteds, Wheat	5	80	
Townhouse Bistro, Corn Bread	2	80	
Townhouse Bistro, low salt	5	80	
Townhouse Bistro, Multigrain	2	80	
Townhouse Bistro, original	5	80	
Townhouse Bistro, reduced fat	6	60	
Townhouse Bistro, Rye	2	70	
Townhouse Bistro, Wheat	5	80	
Wheatables, 7 grain	17	140	
Wheatables, Honey Wheat	17	140	
Wheatable, original	17	140	
Wheatables, reduced fat	19	140	
Zesta, f-f	5	60	
Zesta, original	5	60	

Protein (g)	Total Fat (g)	Sat. Fat (g)	Trans Fat (g)	Chol. (mg)	Sodium (mg)	Calcium (%)	Iron (%)	Carbs (g)	Fiber (g)
4	4	1	0	0	360	4	10	20	<1
2	6	2.5	0	0	280	0	6	20	<1
2	6	2.5	0	0	280	0	8	19	<1
2	8	2.5	0	0	280	0	8	18	<1
1	1.5	0.5	0.5	0	230	0	2	11	<1
1	1.5	0.5	0	0	230	0	2	12	0
1	1.5	0.5	0.5	0	230	0	2	11	<1
1	3.5	1	0	0	150	0	2	10	<1
1	3.5	1	0	0	160	0	2	11	<1
1	3.5	1	0	0	140	0	2	10	<1
1	3.5	1	0	0	160	0	2	10	<1
1	3	0.5	1	5	100	0	2	11	<1
1	4.5	1	0	0	80	0	2	10	<1
1	3	0.5	1	0	130	0	2	11	<1
1	4.5	1	0	0	140	0	2	9	<1
1	1.5	0.5	0	0	160	0	2	11	<1
1	3	0.5	1	0	180	0	2	11	<1
1	4	1	0	0	140	0	2	10	<1
2	6	1.5	0	0	320	0	4	20	1
2	6	1.5	0	0	320	0	4	20	1
2	6	1.5	0	0	300	0	4	20	1
2	4	1	0	0	320	0	6	23	1
1	0	0	0	0	280	0	4	13	<1
1	1.5	0.5	0.5	0	230	0	2	11	<1

Crackers FOOD NAME	Portion Size	Calories	
Zesta, whole grain wheat	5	60	
Nabisco			
Cheese Nips, Cheddar	1 oz	150	
Cheese Nips, Four Cheese	1 oz	150	
Ritz Bits, Cracker Sandwich, Peanut Butter	1 oz	140	
Ritz, Dinosaurs	1 oz	130	
Ritz, original	½ oz	80	
Ritz, reduced fat	½ oz	70	
Ritz, Top'ems	½ oz	70	
Ritz, whole wheat	½ oz	70	
Triscuit, Deli-Style Rye	1 oz	120	
Triscuit, Garden Herb	1 oz	120	
Triscuit, original	1 oz	120	
Triscuit, reduced fat	1 oz	120	
Wheat Thins, Honey	1 oz	150	
Wheat Thins, Multigrain	1 oz	130	
Wheat Thins, original	1 oz	150	
Wheat Thins, Ranch	1 oz	140	
Wheat Thins, reduced fat	1 oz	130	
Old London			
Melba Flatbread Crackers, Sesame	2	60	
Melba JJ Flats, Flavorall	1	60	
Melba JJ Flats, Sesame	1	60	
Melba rounds (12-grain, Vegetable)	5	50	
Melba Snacks (Onion)	5	60	

Protein (g)	Total Fat (g)	Sat. Fat (g)	Trans Fat (g)	Chol. (mg)	Sodium (mg)	Calcium (%)	Iron (%)	Carbs (g)	Fiber (g)
1	1.5	0.5	0.5	0	230	0	2	11	<1
3	7	1.5	0	5	340	2	6	18	1
3	7	1.5	0	0	310	2	6	18	1
3	8	1.5	0	0	240	4	4	16	1
2	4	1	0	0	290	6	6	22	1
1	4	1	0	0	135	2	4	10	0
1	2	0	0	0	150	2	4	11	0
1	3	0.5	0	0	130	2	2	10	0
1	2.5	0.5	0	0	120	2	2	11	1
3	4.5	0.5	0	0	150	0	6	19	3
3	4	0.5	0	0	125	0	8	20	3
3	4.5	0.5	0	0	180	0	8	19	3
3	3	0	0	0	160	0	6	21	3
2	6	1	0	0	260	2	6	21	1
2	4.5	0.5	0	0	230	4	6	22	2
3	6	1	0	0	270	2	6	21	1
2	6	1	0	0	220	2	6	19	1
3	4	0.5	0	0	260	2	6	21	1
2	2	0	0	<5	140	na	na	9	1
2	2.5	0.5	0	<5	150	na	na	9	1
2	2	0	0	<5	140	na	na	9	1
2	0	0	0	0	90	na	na	12	1
2	1.5	0	0	0	140	na	na	12	1

Crackers – Cream / FOOD NAME	Portion Size	Calories	
Melba Toast (White, Garlic, or Wheat)	3	50	
Pepperidge Farm Goldfish			
Baby	89 pcs	140	
Cheddar	55 pcs	140	
Original	55 pcs	150	
Parmesan	60 pcs	130	
Pizza	55 pcs	140	
Pretzel	43 pcs	130	
CRANBERRY			
Dried, sweetened (S&W Craisins)	⅓ c	130	
Fresh, raw	1 c	51	
Sauce, canned, whole berry (S&W)	¼ c	100	
Sauce, canned, jellied (S&W)	¼ c	100	
CRANBERRY BEVERAGES			
Langers, Cranberry Juice Cocktail	8 oz	140	
Langers, Diet Cranberry	8 oz	30	
Langers, White Cranberry	8 oz	120	
Langers, White Cranberry Raspberry	8 oz	120	
Ocean Spray, 100% Cocktail	8 oz	130	
Ocean Spray, Cran-Apple	8 oz	140	
Santa Cruz, Cranberry Nectar, Organic	8 oz	110	
CREAM			
Half & Half	1 oz	39	
Half & Half, f-f	1 oz	18	
Heavy Whipping Cream	1 oz	103	

Protein (g)	Total Fat (g)	Sat. Fat (g)	Trans Fat (g)	Chol. (mg)	Sodium (mg)	Calcium (%)	Iron (%)	Carbs (g)	Fiber (g)
2	0	0	0	0	90	na	na	11	1
4	5	1	0	<5	250	4	4	20	<1
4	5	1	0	<5	250	4	2	20	<1
3	6	0.5	0	0	230	2	4	20	<1
4	4	1	0	0	280	6	6	20	<1
3	6	1	0	0	230	2	8	20	<1
3	2.5	0.5	0	0	430	0	8	24	<1
0	0	0	0	0	0	na	na	33	2
0	0	0	0	0	2	1	2	13	5
0	0	0	0	0	35	0	0	26	1
0	0	0	0	0	35	0	0	26	0
0	0	0	0	0	10	na	na	35	na
0	0	0	0	0	10	na	na	8	na
0	0	0	0	0	10	na	na	28	na
0	0	0	0	0	10	na	na	28	na
0	0	0	0	0	35	0	2	33	0
0	0	0	0	0	80	na	na	35	na
<1	0	0	0	0	25	2	4	27	0
1	3	2	0	11	12	3	0	1	0
1	0	0	0	2	43	3	0	3	0
1	11	7	0	41	11	2	0	1	0

FOOD NAME	Portion Size	Calories	
Light Whipping Cream	1 oz	83	
CREAMERS (COFFEE)			
Coffee-Mate, liquid, Amaretto	1 Tbs	35	
Coffee-Mate, liquid, Chocolate Raspberry	1 Tbs	35	
Coffee-Mate, liquid, Cinnamon Vanilla Crème	1 Tbs	35	
Coffee-Mate, liquid, French Vanilla, f-f	1 Tbs	25	
Coffee-Mate, Latte Creations, half & half Vanilla	1 Tbs	60	
Coffee-Mate, powder, Coconut Crème	4 tsp	60	
Coffee-Mate, powder, Creamy Chocolate	4 tsp	60	
Coffee-Mate, powder, Vanilla Caramel	4 tsp	60	
International Delight, Amaretto	1 Tbs	40	
International Delight, Chocolate Caramel	1 Tbs	45	
International Delight, French Vanilla	1 Tbs	40	
International Delight, Irish Crème, f-f	1 Tbs	30	
CROUTONS			
Mrs. Cubbison's Garlic & Butter	8 pcs	30	
Pepperidge Farm, Classic Caesar	6 pcs	35	
Pepperidge Farm, Four Cheese & Garlic	6 pcs	30	
Pepperidge Farm, Onion & Garlic	6 pcs	30	
Pepperidge Farm, Whole Grain Caesar	6 pcs	35	
Pepperidge Farm, Zesty Italian	6 pcs	30	
CUCUMBER, raw, sliced, peeled	1 c	14	
CURRANTS, raw, red & white	1 c	63	
Zante (Sun-Maid)	¼ c	120	

Protein (g)	Total Fat (g)	Sat. Fat (g)	Trans Fat (g)	Chol. (mg)	Sodium (mg)	Calcium (%)	Iron (%)	Carbs (g)	Fiber (g)
1	9	5	0	31	10	2	0	1	0
0	1.5	0	0	0	10	0	0	5	0
0	1.5	0	0	0	15	0	0	5	0
0	1.5	0	0	0	10	0	0	5	0
0	0	0	0	0	0	0	0	5	0
<1	4	2.5	0	15	80	2	0	7	0
0	3	3	0	0	15	0	0	8	0
0	2.5	2	0	0	30	0	0	9	0
0	3	2.5	0	0	15	0	0	9	0
0	1.5	1	0	0	0	0	0	7	0
0	2	1	0	0	5	0	0	7	0
0	2	1	0	0	5	0	0	7	0
0	0	0	0	0	5	0	0	7	0
0	1	0	na	0	100	0	0	5	0
<1	1.5	0	0	0	55	0	0	5	0
1	1	0	0	0	60	0	0	5	0
<1	1	0	0	0	70	0	0	5	0
1	1	0	0	0	50	0	0	5	0
<1	1	0	0	0	60	0	0	5	0
1	0	0	0	0	2	2	1	3	1
2	0	0	0	0	1	4	6	15	5
1	0	0	0	0	10	2	6	30	2

Dandelion Greens cooked, no salt, chopped – Dips FOOD NAME	Portion Size	Calories	
DANDELION GREENS, cooked,			
no salt, chopped	1 c	35	
DATES, pitted, chopped	1 oz	80	
Pitted (Dole)	¼ c	110	
Pitted (Sun-Maid)	¼ c	120	
DESSERT TOPPINGS			
Cool Whip, Chocolate	2 Tbs	25	
Cool Whip, French Vanilla	2 Tbs	25	
Cool Whip, lite	2 Tbs	20	
Cool Whip, regular	2 Tbs	25	
Cool Whip, sugar free	2 Tbs	20	
Smucker's Butterscotch Caramel	2 Tbs	130	
Smucker's Dove Dark Chocolate	2 Tbs	140	
Smucker's Plate Scrapers Caramel	2 Tbs	100	
Smucker's Plate Scrapers Raspberry	2 Tbs	100	
Smucker's Plate Scrapers Vanilla	2 Tbs	110	
Smucker's Special Recipe Hot Fudge	2 Tbs	140	
DIPS			
Kraft, Bacon & Cheddar	1 oz	60	
Kraft, Creamy Ranch	1 oz	60	
Kraft, French Onion	1 oz	60	
Kraft, Green Onion	1 oz	60	
Kraft, Guacamole	1 oz	50	
Lays, Creamy Ranch	2 Tbs	60	
Lays, French Onion	2 Tbs	50	

Protein (g)	Total Fat (g)	Sat. Fat (g)	Trans Fat (g)	Chol. (mg)	Sodium (mg)	Calcium (%)	Iron (%)	Carbs (g)	Fiber (g)
2	1	0	0	0	46	15	10	7	3
1	0	0	0	0	1	1	2	21	2
1	0	0	0	0	0	2	2	30	4
1	0	0	0	0	10	2	2	33	3
0	1.5	1.5	0	0	0	0	0	2	0
0	1.5	1.5	0	0	0	0	0	2	0
0	1	1	0	0	0	0	0	3	0
0	1.5	1.5	0	0	0	0	0	2	0
0	1	1	0	0	0	0	0	3	0
1	1	0.5	0	<5	70	4	0	30	<1
<1	5	1.5	0	0	80	0	6	22	1
1	0	0	0	0	105	0	0	25	0
0	0	0	0	0	5	0	0	25	0
1	1	0	0	0	0	0	0	24	0
2	4	1	0	0	70	6	4	22	<1
1	5	3.5	0	5	170	0	0	3	0
1	4.5	3	0	0	1990	0	0	3	0
1	4.5	3	0	0	210	0	0	3	0
1	4	3	0	0	190	0	0	4	0
1	4.5	2.5	0	0	240	0	0	3	0
1	5	2.5	0	<5	240	0	0	1	<1
1	5	2	0	<5	230	0	0	2	<1

FOOD NAME	Portion Size	Calories
DOUGHNUTS (also see Fast Food, Dunkin' Donuts)		
Entenmann's, Cinnamon	1	240
Entenmann's Devil's Food	1	310
Entenmann's Devil's Food Crumb	1	260
Entenmann's Plain	1	210
Entenmann's Powdered	1	240
Tastykake, Cinnamon Holes	4	210
Tastykake, Glazed Holes, Blueberry	4	220
Tastykake, Glazed Holes, Chocolate	4	220
Tastykake, Powdered Holes	4	210
DUCK, roasted w/skin, diced	1 c	472
Roasted, without skin, diced	1 c	281
EGGS		
Chicken, whole, raw, large	1	73
Chicken, white only, large	1	17
Chicken, yolk only, large	1	55
Chicken, whole, hard-boiled, large	1	77
Chicken, whole, poached, large	1	73
Duck, whole, fresh	1	129
Goose, whole, fresh	1	266
Quail, whole, fresh	1	14
EGG SUBSTITUTES		
Ener-G-Egg	1½ tsp	15
Morningstar Better 'n Eggs	¼ c	20

Protein (g)	Total Fat (g)	Sat. Fat (g)	Trans Fat (g)	Chol. (mg)	Sodium (mg)	Calcium (%)	Iron (%)	Carbs (g)	Fiber (g)
2	13	7	0	0	230	2	4	28	<1
2	19	6	0	10	180	4	10	36	2
3	13	7	0	10	200	4	6	34	1
2	13	6	0	0	230	2	4	22	<1
2	13	6	0	0	220	2	4	28	<1
3	10	2	3	20	210	2	6	28	<1
2	12	6	4.5	0	190	6	4	27	<1
3	13	7	5	10	220	8	6	26	1
3	10	2	3	20	210	2	6	27	<1
27	40	14	0	118	83	2	21	0	0
33	16	6	0	125	91	2	21	0	0
6	5	2	0	211	70	3	5	0	0
4	0	0	0	0	55	0	0	0	0
3	5	2	0	210	8	2	3	1	0
6	5	2	0	212	62	2	3	1	0
6	5	2	0	211	147	3	5	0	0
9	10	3	0	619	102	4	15	1	0
2	19	5	0	1227	199	9	29	2	0
1	1	0	0	70	13	1	2	0	0
0	0	0	0	0	5	10	0	4	0
5	0	0	0	0	90	2	4	0	0

FOOD NAME	Portion Size	Calories
Morningstar Scramblers	¼ c	35
EGGPLANT, boiled, no salt, cubes	1 c	35
ENDIVE, raw, chopped	1 c	8
FAST FOOD—Arby's		
Arby's Melt Sandwich	1	300
Apple Turnover, no icing	1	250
Bacon Biscuit	1	300
Bacon, Beef & Cheddar Sandwich	1	520
Bacon & Egg Croissant	1	410
Beef & Cheddar Sandwich	1	440
Buttermilk Ranch Dressing	1 pkt	290
Chicken Breast Fillet, Crispy	1	640
Chicken Breast Fillet, Grilled	1	410
Chicken Fingers	3 pack	430
Chicken Fingers	5 pack	720
Chicken Salad Sandwich w/Pecans	1	880
Corned Beef Reuben	1	610
Cool Ranch Sour Cream Dipping Sauce	1 pkt	160
Curly Fries	small	340
Curly Fries	med	410
Curly Fries	large	630
Gourmet Chocolate Cookie	1	200
Honey Mustard Dipping Sauce	1 pkt	130
Hot Ham & Swiss Melt	1	270
Jalapeno Bites, regular	5	310

Protein (g)	Total Fat (g)	Sat. Fat (g)	Trans Fat (g)	Chol. (mg)	Sodium (mg)	Calcium (%)	Iron (%)	Carbs (g)	Fiber (g)
6	0	0	0	0	60	2	6	2	0
1	0	0	0	0	1	1	1	9	2
0	0	0	0	0	10	2	2	2	2
16	12	4.5	1	30	920	6	15	36	2
4	15	4	6	0	200	0	0	35	2
9	17	5	na	15	950	2	80	27	<1
27	27	9	2	65	1570	8	25	45	2
13	26	12	na	190	670	4	15	31	<1
22	21	7	2	50	1270	6	20	44	2
1	5	1	1	25	580	4	0	3	0
36	33	6	1	60	1010	10	15	53	3
32	17	3	0	10	910	8	16	00	3
29	21	5	1	50	1360	25	10	32	2
48	35	9	2	80	2270	45	20	54	4
29	46	7	1	70	1240	20	25	92	7
34	27	7	1	85	1850	35	30	55	3
1	16	4	0	30	280	2	0	2	0
4	20	3.5	3	0	790	4	10	39	4
5	24	4.5	4	0	950	6	10	47	5
8	37	7	6	0	1480	8	20	73	7
2	10	4	2	15	210	2	8	26	<1
0	12	2	1	10	170	0	0	5	0
18	8	3.5	0	35	1140	15	15	35	1
5	21	9	2	30	530	4	6	29	2

FOOD NAME	Portion Size	Calories	
Jr. Roast Beef Sandwich	1	270	
Kids Meal, Chicken Tenders	2 pak	290	
Loaded Potato Bites, small	5	350	
Loaded Potato Bites	10	710	
Onion Petals	regular	330	
Roast Beef	regular	320	
Roast Beef	med	420	
Roast Beef	large	550	
Roast Turkey & Swiss Sandwich	1	720	
Roast turkey, Ranch & Bacon Wrap,	1	700	
Salad: Chicken Club, no dressing	1	500	
Salad: Martha's Vineyard, no dressing	1	270	
Salad: Santa Fe, no dressing	1	490	
Sausage Biscuit	1	390	
Sausage, Egg & Cheese Wrap	1	720	
Shakes: Vanilla, Strawberry, Jamoca	regular	500	
Shakes: Chocolate	regular	510	
Sourdough Bacon, Egg & Swiss Sandwich	1	500	
Super Roast Beef Sandwich	1	400	
Tangy Southwest Sauce	1 pkt	330	
Ultimate BLT Sandwich	1	780	
FAST FOOD—Baskin Robbins			
Banana Nut	½ c	260	
Black Walnut	½ c	280	
Cherries Jubilee	½ c	240	

Protein (g)	Total Fat (g)	Sat. Fat (g)	Trans Fat (g)	Chol. (mg)	Sodium (mg)	Calcium (%)	Iron (%)	Carbs (g)	Fiber (g)
16	9	4	0.5	30	740	6	15	34	2
9	14	3.5	0	30	910	15	8	21	1
11	22	7	2	15	800	20	6	27	2
23	44	14	3	25	1600	35	10	54	5
4	23	4	1	0	330	2	4	35	2
21	14	5	1	45	950	6	20	34	2
31	21	9	1	75	1380	6	25	31	2
42	28	12	2	100	1800	6	35	41	3
45	30	8	1	90	1790	35	30	74	5
49	37	11	1	110	2220	20	30	45	4
33	9	6	1	210	1240	40	20	32	5
26	8	4	0	70	450	20	8	22	4
30	23	9	1	60	1230	40	20	40	6
10	27	9	na	30	1080	2	80	26	<1
24	45	16	na	205	1850	40	20	53	2
13	13	8	0	35	360	50	4	81	0
13	13	8	0	35	360	40	2	83	0
25	29	10	na	325	1600	30	20	33	1
21	19	6	1	45	1060	6	20	41	2
1	35	5	2	30	370	0	0	5	0
23	45	11	1	50	1570	15	25	75	6
5	16	7	0	45	75	15	2	27	1
6	19	9	0	50	90	15	2	25	1
4	12	7	0	45	80	15	2	30	1

Fast Food—Baskin Robbins FOOD NAME	Portion Size	Calories	
Chocolate	½ c	260	
Chocolate Almond	½ c	300	
Chocolate Chip Cookie Dough	½ c	290	
Chocolate Chip	½ c	270	
Chocolate Fudge	½ c	270	
Chocolate Oreo	½ c	330	
French Vanilla	½ c	280	
Fudge Brownie	½ c	300	
German Chocolate Cake	½ c	300	
Jamoca	½ c	240	
Mint Chocolate Chip	½ c	270	
Nutty Coconut	½ c	300	
Old Fashioned Butter Pecan	½ c	280	
Oreo Cookies 'n Cream	½ c	280	
Peanut Butter & Chocolate	½ c	320	
Pistachio Almond	½ c	290	
Pralines 'n Cream	½ c	270	
Rocky Road	½ c	290	
Vanilla	½ c	260	
Very Berry Strawberry	½ c	220	
Low-Fat, No Sugar Added Ice Cream			
Berries & Bananas	½ c	110	
Blueberry Swirl	½ c	130	
Caramel Turtle	½ c	160	
Chocolate Chip	½ c	170	

Protein (g)	Total Fat (g)	Sat. Fat (g)	Trans Fat (g)	Chol. (mg)	Sodium (mg)	Calcium (%)	Iron (%)	Carbs (g)	Fiber (g)
5	14	9	0	50	130	15	4	33	0
7	18	9	0	45	120	15	6	32	1
5	15	9	1	55	130	15	2	36	1
5	16	10	0	55	95	15	4	28	1
4	15	10	0	50	140	10	6	35	0
5	19	8	1	40	180	15	6	39	1
4	18	11	0.5	120	85	15	2	26	0
5	19	11	0	45	140	10	6	35	1
5	16	9	0	45	150	15	6	36	1
5	13	9	0	55	90	16	0	26	0
5	16	10	0	55	95	15	4	28	0
6	20	9	0	45	90	16	4	28	0
5	18	9	0	50	150	15	4	24	1
5	15	8	1	50	150	15	4	32	1
7	20	9	0	45	180	15	4	31	1
7	19	9	0	50	85	15	2	25	1
4	14	8	0	45	170	15	2	34	0
5	15	8	0	45	120	15	4	36	1
4	16	10	0.5	65	70	15	0	26	0
4	11	7	0	40	70	15	2	28	0
5	2	1	0	10	125	15	2	25	1
4	2	1	0	10	140	15	0	31	1
5	4	3	0	10	130	15	2	37	0
4	4.5	3.5	0	10	110	15	15	30	1

FOOD NAME	Portion Size	Calories	
Tin Roof Sundae	½ c	189	
Sundaes			
2-Scoop Hot Fudge Sundae	1	530	
3-Scoop Hot Fudge Sundae	1	750	
Banana Royale	1	630	
Banana Split	1	1030	
Happy Camper Waffle Cone Sundae	1	820	
Nonfat soft serve yogurt, no sugar added			
Butter Pecan	½ c	90	
Café Mocha	½ c	90	
Chocolate	½ c	80	
Strawberry Patch	½ c	90	
Vanilla	½ c	90	
Sherbet			
Blue Raspberry	½ c	160	
Rock & Pop	½ c	190	
Twisted Chip	½ c	180	
Wild & Reckless Spirit	½ c	160	
FAST FOOD—Boston Market			
Meals & Sandwiches			
Beef Meatloaf	7.6 oz	480	
Boston Chicken Carver Sandwich	1	690	
Boston Sirloin Dip Carver sandwich	1	920	
Boston Turkey Carver Sandwich	1	830	
Chicken, 3 Piece Dark, individual meal	1 meal	390	

Protein (g)	Total Fat (g)	Sat. Fat (g)	Trans Fat (g)	Chol. (mg)	Sodium (mg)	Calcium (%)	Iron (%)	Carbs (g)	Fiber (g)
4	3	1.5	0	10	105	15	0	34	1
8	29	19	0	85	200	20	2	62	0
11	41	27	0	125	280	30	2	86	0
9	27	16	0	85	250	25	6	91	5
12	39	23	0	135	190	35	6	168	7
17	41	18	0.5	65	490	20	10	107	5
4	0	0	0	5	90	15	0	17	1
4	0	0	0	5	85	15	0	18	1
4	0	0	0	0	80	15	2	15	0
4	0	0	0	5	85	15	0	17	1
4	0	0	0	5	85	15	0	17	1
1	2	1.5	0	10	40	4	2	34	0
1	4	3	0	10	45	4	0	37	0
1	3	2	0	10	35	4	2	36	0
1	2	1.5	0	10	40	6	0	33	0
29	33	13	0	125	970	na	na	23	2
48	32	7	0	120	14	na	na	96	6
64	43	12	7	200	1260	na	na	70	3
57	35	8	0	90	1810	na	na	70	3
43	20	6	0	220	480	na	na	3	0

FOOD NAME	Portion Size	Calories	
Chicken, Dark Rotisserie, no skin	¼ bird	260	
Chicken, White Rotisserie, no skin	¼ bird	250	
Chicken Pot Pie	1	800	
Meatloaf Carver Sandwich	1	940	
Roasted Turkey	5 oz	180	
Sides & Desserts			
Apple Pie	1 slice	420	
Butternut Squash	1 serv	140	
Chicken Tortilla Soup w/toppings	1 serv	340	
Chocolate Cake	1 slice	600	
Chocolate Chip Fudge Brownie	1	580	
Chocolate Fudge Bliss	1	300	
Cinnamon Apple	1	210	
Corn	1 serv	170	
Garlic Dill Potatoes	1 serv	140	
Macaroni & Cheese	1 serv	330	
Mashed Potatoes w/Gravy	1 serv	235	
Spinach w/Garlic Butter	1 serv	130	
Strawberry Bliss	1	370	
Sweet Potato Casserole	1	460	
Vegetable Stuffing	1 serv	190	
FAST FOOD—Burger King			
Angus Steak Burger	1	560	
Bacon Cheeseburger	1	370	
BK Big Fish	1	630	

Protein (g)	Total Fat (g)	Sat. Fat (g)	Trans Fat (g)	Chol. (mg)	Sodium (mg)	Calcium (%)	Iron (%)	Carbs (g)	Fiber (g)
30	13	4	0	155	260	na	na	2	0
41	8	2.5	0	126	480	na	na	4	0
29	49	18	0	115	800	na	na	59	4
49	45	18	0	155	2080	na	na	96	6
38	3	1	0	70	620	na	na	70	3
3	20	4	5	0	650	na	na	56	2
2	4.5	3	0	10	35	na	na	25	2
12	22	7	0	45	1310	na	na	24	1
5	32	7	4.5	65	210	na	na	75	2
9	23	5	na	90	390	na	na	81	3
4	8	6	0	25	210	na	na	58	2
0	3	0	0	0	15	na	na	47	3
6	4	1	0	95	37	na	na	37	2
3	3	1	0	0	120	na	na	24	3
14	12	7	0.5	30	1290	na	na	39	1
5	10	6	0	25	960	na	na	32	3
5	9	6	0	20	200	na	na	9	5
3	23	10	0	90	190	na	na	37	0
4	17	6	0	20	210	na	na	77	3
3	8	1	0	0	580	na	na	25	2
33	22	8	1.5	180	1190	10	35	59	3
20	19	8	0.5	50	920	15	20	31	1
24	30	6	2.5	60	1380	10	25	67	4

Fast Food—Burger King

FOOD NAME	Portion Size	Calories
BK Big Fish, w/o Tartar Sauce	1	470
BK Chicken Fries	9 pcs	470
BK Veggie Burger	1	420
Cheeseburger	1	330
Chicken Tenders	8 pcs	340
Croissan'wich w/Ham, Egg, Cheese	1	340
Double Croissan'wich w/Double Sausage	1	680
Double Whopper	1	900
Double Whopper w/Cheese	1	990
Dutch Apple Pie	1	300
Enormous Omelet Sandwich	1	740
French Fries, salted	med	360
French Fries, unsalted	med	360
French Toast Sticks	5	390
Garden Salad, side	1	20
Hamburger	1	290
Hash Browns	1 serv	230
Icee Cherry	med	140
Low-carb Angus Steak Burger	1	260
Minute Maid Orange Juice	1	140
Onion Rings	med	320
Original Chicken Sandwich	1	660
Shake, Chocolate	med	690
Shake, Strawberry	med	660
Shake, Vanilla	med	560

Protein (g)	Total Fat (g)	Sat. Fat (g)	Trans Fat (g)	Chol. (mg)	Sodium (mg)	Calcium (%)	Iron (%)	Carbs (g)	Fiber (g)
23	13	3	2	50	1240	10	20	65	3
19	31	6	4.5	55	1350	2	9	20	3
23	4.5	2.5	0	10	1100	15	25	46	7
17	16	7	0.5	55	780	15	15	31	1
19	29	5	3	55	960	2	5	21	<1
18	18	6	2	160	1510	15	15	26	<1
29	51	18	3	220	1600	15	0	26	<1
47	57	19	2	175	1090	15	45	51	3
52	64	24	2.5	195	1520	30	45	52	3
2	13	3	3	0	270	0	6	45	1
36	46	17	1	330	2080	30	35	45	3
4	20	4.5	4.5	0	590	2	4	41	4
4	20	4.5	4.5	0	380	2	4	41	4
7	20	4.5	4.5	0	440	6	10	46	2
1	0	0	0	0	15	0	2	4	<1
15	12	4.5	0.5	40	560	8	15	30	1
2	15	4	5	0	450	0	2	23	2
0	0	0	0	0	10	0	0	40	0
24	18	7	1	180	490	2	15	2	<1
2	0	0	0	0	25	0	0	33	0
4	16	4	3.5	0	480	10	0	40	3
24	40	8	2.5	70	1440	10	20	52	4
11	20	12	0	75	560	45	10	114	2
10	19	12	0	75	330	45	2	111	0
11	21	13	0.5	85	330	50	2	79	0

FOOD NAME	Portion Size	Calories	
Tendercrisp Chicken Sandwich	1	780	
Tendercrisp Caesar Salad	1	400	
Tendercrisp Garden Salad	1	410	
Tendergrill Chicken Sandwich	1	450	
Tendergrill Garden Salad	1	230	
Triple Whopper Sandwich	1	1130	
Triple Whopper Sandwich w/ Cheese	1	1230	
Whopper Sandwich	1	670	
Whopper Jr. Sandwich	1	370	
Whopper Jr. Sandwich w/ Cheese	1	410	
FAST FOOD—Church's Chicken			
Apple Pie	1	260	
Cajun Rice	regular	130	
Chicken Fried Steak Sandwich	1	490	
Chicken Fried Steak w/ Gravy	2 pcs	610	
Cole Slaw	regular	150	
Double Lemon Pie	1	300	
French Fries	regular	420	
Jalapeno Bombers	4	240	
Maccaroni & Cheese	regular	210	
Mashed Potatoes w/ Gravy	regular	70	
Okra	regular	300	
Original Breast	1 pc	200	
Original Leg	1 pc	110	
Original Tender Strip	1 pc	120	

Protein (g)	Total Fat (g)	Sat. Fat (g)	Trans Fat (g)	Chol. (mg)	Sodium (mg)	Calcium (%)	Iron (%)	Carbs (g)	Fiber (g)
26	43	8	4	75	1730	10	20	73	4
23	21	5	3.5	55	1240	20	10	31	3
24	21	6	3.5	55	1250	20	10	34	4
37	10	2	0	75	1210	8	25	53	4
32	8	3	0	60	720	20	15	11	3
67	74	27	3	255	1160	15	60	52	3
71	82	32	3.5	275	1590	30	60	52	3
28	39	11	1.5	95	1020	15	30	51	3
15	21	6	0.5	50	560	8	15	31	2
18	24	8	1	60	780	15	20	32	2
2	11	4	2	5	250	0	8	39	1
1	7	3	0	5	260	0	15	16	<5
13	32	8	2	30	880	6	18	38	2
24	43	13	4	70	1465	4	16	31	2
1	10	2	0	5	170	2	2	15	2
6	14	6	0	25	160	10	4	39	0
5	20	6	6	5	450	4	14	55	6
8	10	6	0	30	970	20	3	29	3
8	11	4	0	15	690	12	3	23	1
2	2	0	0	<1	480	2	2	12	1
4	23	4	0	0	740	11	8	27	6
22	11	3	2	80	450	0	6	3	1
10	6	2	1	55	280	0	4	3	0
12	6	2	1	35	44	0	2	6	<1

FOOD NAME	Portion Size	Calories	
Original Thigh	1 pc	330	
Original Wing	1 pc	300	
Spicy Chicken Sandwich	1	360	
Spicy Fish Sandwich	1	320	
Spicy Popcorn Chicken	regular	430	
Spicy Tender Strips	1 pc	135	
Strawberry Cream Cheese Pie	1 pie	280	
FAST FOOD—Dairy Queen			
Desserts, Beverages			
Blizzard, Banana Split	small	460	
Blizzard, Banana Split	med	580	
Blizzard, Banana Split	large	810	
Blizzard, Chocolate Chip Cookie Dough	small	720	
Blizzard, Chocolate Chip Cookie Dough	med	1030	
Blizzard, Chocolate Chip Cookie Dough	large	1320	
Blizzard, Oreo Cookies	small	570	
Blizzard, Oreo Cookies	med	700	
Blizzard, Oreo Cookies	large	1010	
Buster Bar	1	450	
Chocolate Dilly Bar	1	210	
Classic Banana Split	1	510	
Curly Shake, Chocolate	small	620	
Curly Shake, Chocolate	large	1200	
Curly Shake, Strawberry	small	540	
Curly Shake, Strawberry	large	500	

Protein (g)	Total Fat (g)	Sat. Fat (g)	Trans Fat (g)	Chol. (mg)	Sodium (mg)	Calcium (%)	Iron (%)	Carbs (g)	Fiber (g)
21	23	6	3	110	680	2	6	8	1
27	19	5	3	120	540	2	8	7	3
14	18	4	1.5	30	660	8	10	35	3
10	20	4	3	25	560	4	0	25	2
21	23	4	2	50	980	2	8	33	2
11	7	2	2	25	480	0	2	7	4
4	15	8	0	15	130	4	4	32	2
10	14	9	0	40	210	35	8	73	<1
12	17	11	0.5	50	260	40	10	97	1
17	20	15	1	70	360	60	15	134	2
12	28	14	2.5	60	670	55	15	105	0
17	40	20	4	70	520	45	20	150	0
21	52	26	5	90	670	60	25	193	0
11	21	10	2.5	40	430	35	15	83	<1
13	26	12	4	45	560	40	15	103	1
19	37	18	5	70	770	60	25	148	2
10	28	12	1	15	280	15	6	41	2
3	13	7	0	10	75	10	2	21	0
8	12	8	0	30	180	25	10	96	3
13	18	11	0.5	55	300	45	10	102	1
26	34	22	1	103	570	90	15	197	2
13	17	11	0.5	55	270	45	10	85	<1
10	15	9	0	45	230	40	10	83	<1

FOOD NAME	Portion Size	Calories	
DQ Fudge Bar	1	50	
DQ Vanilla Orange Bar	1	60	
Misty, Cherry	small	210	
Misty, Cherry	large	430	
Misty, Grape	small	240	
Misty, Grape	large	480	
Misty, Lemon Lime	small	140	
Misty, Lemon Lime	large	280	
Peanut Butter Blast	1	700	
Pecan Praline Parfait	1	720	
Starkiss Bar	1	80	
Strawberry Shortcake	1	430	
Sundae, Chocolate	small	280	
Sundae, Chocolate	large	580	
Sundae, Strawberry	small	240	
Sundae, Strawberry	large	500	
Vanilla Cone	small	230	
Vanilla Cone	med	330	
Vanilla Cone	large	480	
Sandwiches, Sides			
Bacon Cheeseburger	1	750	
Buffalo Chicken Strips	4 strips	540	
Buttermilk Dressing, reduced calorie	1 pkt	140	
California Grillburger	1	690	
Chicken Quesadilla	1	550	

Protein (g)	Total Fat (g)	Sat. Fat (g)	Trans Fat (g)	Chol. (mg)	Sodium (mg)	Calcium (%)	Iron (%)	Carbs (g)	Fiber (g)
4	0	0	0	0	70	10	0	13	0
2	0	0	0	0	40	6	0	17	0
0	0	0	0	0	15	0	0	58	0
0	0	0	0	0	30	0	0	116	0
0	0	0	0	0	20	0	0	66	0
0	0	0	0	0	35	0	0	132	0
0	0	0	0	0	110	0	0	38	0
0	0	0	0	0	220	0	0	76	0
12	37	19	0	35	380	25	6	79	2
9	29	11	0.5	30	610	30	6	105	1
0	0	0	0	0	10	0	0	21	0
7	14	9	1	60	360	25	10	70	1
5	7	4.5	0	20	110	20	4	40	0
10	15	10	0	45	260	35	10	100	1
5	7	4.5	0	20	110	20	4	40	0
10	15	9	0	45	230	40	10	83	<1
6	7	4.5	0	20	115	20	6	38	0
8	9	6	0	30	160	25	10	53	0
11	15	9	0.5	45	230	35	15	76	0
37	46	19	4	125	1470	20	20	47	<1
31	30	6	6	65	2560	4	20	36	3
0	13	2	0	15	390	2	0	5	0
28	44	13	4	100	730	8	15	43	0
32	31	17	2	90	1160	45	15	35	3

FOOD NAME	Portion Size	Calories	
Chicken Strips, no sauce	4 strips	400	
Classic Grillburger, no cheese	1	600	
Classic Hot Dog	1	400	
Classic Hot Dog, Chili Cheese	1	510	
Crispy Chicken Salad, no dressing or croutons	1	350	
Crispy Chicken Sandwich	1	6900	
DQ Honey Mustard Dressing	1 pkt	260	
Fish Fillets, no sauce	4	440	
French Fries	5 oz	380	
French Fries	7 oz	530	
Grilled Chicken Salad	1	240	
Grilled Chicken Sandwich	1	520	
Grilled Turkey Sandwich	1	730	
Half lb. Grillburger, no cheese	1	860	
House Salad, no dressing or croutons	1	120	
Onion Rings	4 oz	470	
Onion Rings	5 oz	590	
Vegetable Quesadilla	1	440	
FAST FOOD—Dunkin' Donuts			
Bagels			
Cinnamon raisin	1	330	
Everything	1	370	
Multigrain	1	380	
Plain	1	320	

Protein (g)	Total Fat (g)	Sat. Fat (g)	Trans Fat (g)	Chol. (mg)	Sodium (mg)	Calcium (%)	Iron (%)	Carbs (g)	Fiber (g)
26	24	4.5	5	40	740	2	8	21	4
28	33	12	3	90	1100	8	20	48	<1
15	27	11	1.5	55	1190	8	15	26	1
21	35	15	2	75	1400	20	20	29	2
21	20	6	2.5	40	620	15	10	21	6
22	37	6	4	65	1260	10	25	64	2
1	21	3.5	0	20	370	2	6	18	0
18	24	8	5	40	1020	0	8	40	0
4	15	3	4	0	880	2	6	56	4
6	21	4	6	0	1225	4	8	78	6
26	10	5	0	65	950	15	8	12	4
25	26	4.5	2	80	1190	6	6	44	0
33	45	10	5	95	1770	15	120	45	<1
49	53	21	5	155	1340	10	30	48	<1
6	5	3	0	15	125	15	8	12	4
6	30	6	7	0	740	2	8	45	3
7	37	7	9	0	930	4	8	56	4
20	25	13	2	55	690	45	15	34	3
10	3	0.5	0	0	430	4	20	65	3
14	6	0.5	0	0	650	6	25	67	3
14	6	1	0	0	650	4	30	68	5
12	2.5	0.5	0	0	650	0	20	62	2

Fast Food—Dunkin' Donuts FOOD NAME	Portion Size	Calories	
Sesame	1	380	
Wheat	1	330	
Bakery			
Apple Danish	1	330	
Banana Walnut Muffin	1	540	
Biscuit	1	250	
Blueberry Muffin	1	470	
Cheese Danish	1	340	
Chocolate Chip Muffin	1	630	
Chocolate Chunk Cookie	2	220	
Chocolate Chunk Cookie w/ Walnuts	2	230	
Coffee Cake Muffin	1	580	
Corn Muffin	1	510	
Oatmeal Raisin Pecan Cookie	2	220	
Plain Croissant	1	330	
Beverages			
Cappuccino w/soy	10 oz	70	
Caramel Crème Latte	10 oz	260	
Caramel Swirl Latte, w/ soy	10 oz	210	
Coffee Coolatta, w/ 2% milk	16 oz	190	
Coffee Coolatta, w/ cream	16 oz	350	
Dunkaccino	10 oz	230	
Espresso	2 oz	0	
Flavored Coffees, all	10 oz	20	
Hot Latte, lite	10 oz	70	

Protein (g)	Total Fat (g)	Sat. Fat (g)	Trans Fat (g)	Chol. (mg)	Sodium (mg)	Calcium (%)	Iron (%)	Carbs (g)	Fiber (g)
14	8	0.5	0	0	650	0	20	64	3
12	4	1	0	0	610	0	20	62	4
4	20	9	0	30	260	0	6	32	1
10	25	3.5	0	65	520	6	15	89	3
5	13	3.5	8	0	780	4	8	29	1
8	17	3	0	60	500	4	15	73	2
4	22	10	0	35	280	2	6	30	1
10	26	8	0	70	560	4	15	89	2
3	11	7	0	35	105	0	4	28	1
3	12	6	0	35	110	0	4	27	1
9	19	3	0	65	520	4	15	78	1
8	18	3.5	0	75	860	2	15	77	1
3	10	5	0	30	110	0	4	29	1
5	18	4.5	7	5	270	0	0	37	5
4	2.5	0	0	0	80	20	4	6	1
8	9	6	0	20	125	30	0	40	0
8	3.5	0	0	0	160	35	6	34	1
4	2	1.5	0	10	80	15	0	41	0
3	22	14	0	75	65	10	0	40	0
2	10	3	5	5	210	4	0	35	0
0	0	0	0	0	5	0	0	1	0
1	0	0	0	0	60-65	0	0	4	0
6	0	0	0	5	80	20	0	10	0

FOOD NAME	Portion Size	Calories	
Iced Coffee w/ cream	16 oz	70	
Iced Coffee w/ skim milk & sugar	16 oz	70	
Iced Latte w/ skim milk	16 oz	70	
Latte w/ soy milk	10 oz	90	
Mocha Almond Iced Latte	16 oz	290	
Tropicana Orange Coolatta	16 oz	370	
Turbo Hot Latte	10 oz	130	
Turbo Ice	16 oz	120	
Vanilla Bean Coolatta	16 oz	440	
Vanilla Chai	10 oz	230	
Cream Cheese			
Chive	2 oz	170	
Garden vegetable	2 oz	170	
Lite	2 oz	110	
Salmon	2 oz	170	
Strawberry	2 oz	190	
Donuts and Fancies			
Apple Crumb	1	230	
Apple Fritter	1	300	
Apple & Spice	1	200	
Bavarian Kreme	1	210	
Blueberry Cake	1	290	
Boston Kreme	1	240	
Chocolate Frosted Cake	1	360	
Chocolate Frosted Donut	1	200	

Protein (g)	Total Fat (g)	Sat. Fat (g)	Trans Fat (g)	Chol. (mg)	Sodium (mg)	Calcium (%)	Iron (%)	Carbs (g)	Fiber (g)
2	6	3.5	0	20	75	4	0	4	0
2	0	0	0	0	75	4	0	16	0
7	0	0	0	0	110	0	0	11	0
6	3.5	0	0	0	110	25	6	8	1
8	10	7	0	20	115	20	8	46	1
1	0	0	0	0	50	0	4	92	3
1	6	3.5	0	20	55	4	0	20	0
1	7	3.5	0	20	25	4	0	14	0
1	17	15	1	0	95	4	0	70	1
1	8	6	0	5	50	2	4	40	0
4	17	11	0	45	230	8	0	4	2
2	15	11	0	45	340	4	0	4	0
4	9	7	0	30	230	4	0	6	0
4	17	11	0	45	180	20	0	2	0
4	17	9	0	45	150	4	0	9	0
3	10	3	0.5	0	270	0	4	34	1
4	14	3	2.5	0	360	0	6	41	1
3	8	1.5	2.5	0	270	0	4	29	1
3	9	2	2.5	0	270	0	4	30	1
3	16	3.5	2.5	10	400	0	6	35	1
3	9	2	3.5	0	280	0	4	36	1
4	20	5	5	25	350	2	8	40	1
3	9	2	5	0	260	0	4	29	1

Fast Food—Dunkin' Donuts FOOD NAME	Portion Size	Calories
Chocolate Glazed Cake	1	290
Chocolate Iced Bismark	1	340
Chocolate Kreme Filled	1	270
Cinnamon Cake Donut	1	330
Cinnamon Cake stick	1	450
Cinnamon Cake Munchkins	4	270
Coffee Roll	1	270
Éclair	1	270
French Cruller	1	150
Glazed Cake Munchkins	3	280
Glazed Cake Stick	1	490
Glazed Chocolate Cake Stick	1	470
Glazed Donut	1	180
Glazed Fritter	1	260
Glazed Lemon Cake	1	240
Jelly Filled Donut	1	210
Jelly Filled Munchkins	5	210
Jelly Filled Sticks	1	530
Lemon Filled Munchkins	4	170
Maple Frosted Donut	1	210
Old Fashioned Cake Donut	1	300
Plain Cake Munchkins	4	270
Plain Cake Stick	1	420
Powdered Cake Donut	1	330
Powdered Cake Stick	1	450

Protein (g)	Total Fat (g)	Sat. Fat (g)	Trans Fat (g)	Chol. (mg)	Sodium (mg)	Calcium (%)	Iron (%)	Carbs (g)	Fiber (g)
3	16	3.5	4	0	370	0	0	33	1
3	15	3.5	1.5	0	290	0	4	50	1
3	13	3	4	0	260	0	4	35	1
4	20	5	4	25	310	2	10	34	1
4	29	7	5	0	490	4	10	49	2
3	15	3.5	4	25	210	2	25	31	1
4	14	3	0	0	340	0	6	33	1
3	11	2.5	0.5	0	290	0	4	39	1
2	8	2	3	20	105	0	0	17	1
3	13	3	4	20	190	0	25	38	1
4	29	7	5	35	310	2	35	51	1
4	29	7	5	0	490	4	10	49	2
3	8	1.5	4	0	250	0	4	25	1
4	14	3	2.5	0	330	0	6	31	1
2	14	3.5	2.5	0	150	0	2	28	0
3	8	1.5	4	0	280	0	4	32	1
3	9	2	2.5	0	240	0	4	30	1
4	29	7	5	35	320	2	35	61	1
2	8	1.5	2.5	0	190	0	0	23	0
3	9	2	2.5	0	260	0	4	30	1
4	19	5	4	25	330	2	8	28	1
3	16	4	4	25	240	0	30	27	1
4	29	7	5	35	310	2	35	35	1
4	19	5	4	25	330	2	8	36	1
4	29	7	5	35	310	2	35	42	1

FOOD NAME	Portion Size	Calories	
Sugar Raised Donut	1	170	
Sugar Raised Munchkins	7	170	
Vanilla Crème Filled	1	270	
Sandwiches			
Bacon Cheese Bagel	1	540	
Bacon Egg Cheese Croissant	1	520	
Egg Cheese Bagel	1	470	
Ham Cheese Bagel	1	510	
Ham Egg Cheese Croissant	1	520	
Ham Egg Cheese English Muffin	1	310	
Meatball Panini	1	480	
Sausage Egg Cheese Croissant	1	690	
Steak Panini	1	450	
Southwestern Chicken Panini	1	420	
Supreme Omelet Croissant	1	590	
FAST FOOD—Jack in the Box			
Breakfast			
Bacon, Egg, Cheese Biscuit	1	430	
Breakfast Jack	1	290	
Chicken Biscuit	1	450	
Extreme Sausage Sandwich	1	670	
Meaty Breakfast Burrito	1	480	
Sausage Biscuit	1	440	
Sausage, Egg, Cheese Biscuit	1	740	
Sourdough Breakfast Sandwich	1	420	

Protein (g)	Total Fat (g)	Sat. Fat (g)	Trans Fat (g)	Chol. (mg)	Sodium (mg)	Calcium (%)	Iron (%)	Carbs (g)	Fiber (g)
3	8	1.5	0.5	0	250	0	4	22	1
4	12	2.5	0.5	0	290	0	4	26	1
3	13	3	3.5	0	250	0	4	36	1
18	18	7	0	200	1400	10	35	69	2
16	33	10	7	215	1010	10	15	40	0
20	15	6	0	190	1120	10	35	65	2
26	16	6	0	200	1390	10	35	65	2
20	32	10	7	205	1010	10	15	40	0
21	10	5	0	160	1270	15	30	34	1
22	19	9	0	40	1180	10	20	56	3
22	51	17	7	230	1000	10	15	40	0
30	12	5	0.5	45	1630	20	30	56	3
23	10	5	0	45	970	15	20	57	3
21	38	13	6	260	1040	15	15	42	1
17	25	8	5	220	1100	na	na	34	1
17	12	4.5	0	220	760	na	na	29	1
15	24	6	6	30	980	na	na	42	2
29	48	17	1.5	290	1300	na	na	31	2
25	29	10	1	350	1210	na	na	29	2
12	29	8	5	35	870	na	na	32	2
27	55	17	6	280	1430	na	na	35	2
20	24	8	2	230	980	na	na	31	2

Fast Food—Jack in the Box FOOD NAME	Portion Size	Calories	
Ultimate Breakfast Sandwich	1	570	
Salads & Sides			
Asian Chicken Salad	1	140	
Bacon Cheddar Potato Wedges	1 serv	720	
Beef Monster Taco	1	240	
Chicken Club Salad	1	300	
Natural Cut Fries	small	270	
Natural Cut Fries	large	530	
Onion Rings	8	500	
Seasoned Curly Fries	small	270	
Seasoned Curly Fries	large	550	
Stuffed Jalapenos	7	530	
Sandwiches, Entrées			
Bacon Bacon Cheeseburger	1	840	
Bacon Chicken Sandwich	1	440	
Bacon Ultimate Cheeseburger	1	1090	
Chicken Breast Strips	4 strips	500	
Fish 'n' Chips	small	570	
Fish 'n' Chips	large	830	
Hamburger	1	310	
Hamburger w/ Cheese	1	350	
Jumbo Jack	1	600	
Jumbo Jack w/ Cheese	1	690	
Original Ciabatta Burger	1	710	
Sourdough Grilled Chicken Club	1	530	

Protein (g)	Total Fat (g)	Sat. Fat (g)	Trans Fat (g)	Chol. (mg)	Sodium (mg)	Calcium (%)	Iron (%)	Carbs (g)	Fiber (g)
34	27	10	1	445	1700	na	na	49	2
14	1	0	0	25	470	na	na	19	5
21	48	15	12	45	1360	na	na	20	3
8	14	5	2	20	390	na	na	20	3
27	15	6	0	65	880	na	na	13	4
4	12	3	3.5	0	440	na	na	35	3
8	25	6	7	0	870	na	na	69	5
6	30	6	10	0	420	na	na	51	3
4	15	3	5	0	590	na	na	30	3
8	31	6	10	0	1200	na	na	60	6
15	30	13	4.5	45	1600	na	na	51	4
34	56	19	1.5	95	1610	na	na	51	2
19	24	6	2.5	40	970	na	na	39	2
46	77	30	3	140	2040	na	na	53	2
35	25	6	6	80	1260	na	na	36	3
17	30	7	9	35	1100	na	na	58	4
21	42	10	12	35	1530	na	na	92	6
16	14	6	1	40	600	na	na	30	1
18	17	8	1	50	790	na	na	31	1
21	35	12	1.5	45	940	na	na	51	3
25	42	16	1.5	70	1310	na	na	54	3
25	40	12	1.5	55	1200	na	na	64	4
36	28	7	2	85	1430	na	na	34	3

FOOD NAME	Portion Size	Calories	
Sourdough Jack	1	710	
Desserts, Shakes			
Cheesecake	1 serv	310	
Chocolate Ice Cream Shake	16 oz	880	
Oreo Cookie Ice Cream Shake	16 oz	910	
Strawberry Ice Cream Shake	16 oz	880	
Vanilla Ice Cream Shake	16 oz	790	
FAST FOOD—KFC			
Sandwiches, Entrées			
Chicken Pot Pie	1	770	
Crispy Strips	3	400	
Crispy Twists Sandwich	1	670	
Double Crunch Sandwich	1	530	
KFC Snacker	1	320	
KFC Snacker Sandwich, Buffalo	1	260	
KFC Snacker Sandwich, Fish	1	270	
KFC Snacker, Ultimate Cheese	1	280	
Oven Roasted Chicken, breast	1	380	
Oven Roasted Chicken, drumstick	1	140	
Oven Roasted Chicken, thigh	1	360	
Oven Roasted Chicken, whole wing	1	150	
Popcorn Chicken, individual	1	380	
Popcorn Chicken, kids size	1	270	
Popcorn Chicken	large	380	
Sides, Desserts			

Protein (g)	Total Fat (g)	Sat. Fat (g)	Trans Fat (g)	Chol. (mg)	Sodium (mg)	Calcium (%)	Iron (%)	Carbs (g)	Fiber (g)
27	51	18	3	75	1230	na	na	36	3
7	16	9	1	55	220	na	na	34	0
14	45	31	2	135	330	na	na	107	1
14	49	32	2	135	420	na	na	102	1
13	44	31	2	135	290	na	na	105	0
13	44	31	2	135	280	na	na	83	0
33	40	15	14	115	1680	0	20	70	5
29	24	5	4.5	75	1250	0	10	17	0
27	38	7	4	60	1650	15	15	55	3
27	28	6	3	55	1240	8	15	42	3
14	16	3	1.5	25	700	6	15	31	2
14	8	2	1.5	25	870	4	10	32	2
13	10	2	1	25	540	6	10	34	2
15	11	2.5	2	25	790	4	10	32	1
40	19	6	2.5	145	1150	0	6	11	0
14	8	2	1	75	440	0	4	4	0
22	25	7	1.5	165	1060	0	6	12	0
11	9	2.5	1	60	370	0	2	5	0
24	21	5	4.5	75	1250	0	10	17	0
15	16	3.5	3.5	40	850	2	6	16	1
24	21	5	4.5	60	1200	4	10	23	0

FOOD NAME	Portion Size	Calories	
Apple Pie Minis	3	400	
Apple Pie	slice	290	
Baked Beans	1 serv	230	
Baked Cheetos	1 serv	120	
Biscuit	1	190	
Fiery Buffalo Wings	6	440	
HBBQ Wings	6	540	
Hot Wings	6	450	
Little Bucket Chocolate Cream	1	270	
Little Bucket Fudge Brownie	1	270	
Little Bucket Lemon Crème	1	400	
Little Bucket Strawberry Shortcake	1	200	
Mashed Potatoes w/Gravy	1 serv	130	
Potato Wedges	1 serv	240	
Seasoned Rice	1 serv	150	
Sweet n' Spicy Wings	6	460	
Sweet Potato Pie	1 slice	340	
FAST FOOD—McDonald's			
Beverages & Desserts			
Apple Dippers w/dip	1 serv	100	
Chocolate Triple Thick Shake	16 oz	580	
Deluxe Warm Cinnamon Bun	1	590	
Fruit Yogurt Parfait	1	160	
McDonaldland Cookies	2 oz	250	
McFlurry w/M&M's	1	620	

Protein (g)	Total Fat (g)	Sat. Fat (g)	Trans Fat (g)	Chol. (mg)	Sodium (mg)	Calcium (%)	Iron (%)	Carbs (g)	Fiber (g)
1	22	5	7	0	70	0	2	22	1
2	11	3	2.5	0	230	2	4	44	2
8	1	1	0	0	720	15	30	30	15
2	4.5	1	0	0	210	0	4	17	0
2	10	2	3.5	15	580	0	4	23	0
27	26	7	3.5	155	1800	4	8	26	3
25	33	7	4.5	150	1130	6	15	36	1
24	29	6	4	145	1120	8	10	23	1
2	13	8	0.5	0	180	2	6	37	2
2	9	4	0.5	30	170	4	4	44	1
4	14	7	1.5	5	210	20	0	65	2
2	6	4	0	20	110	2	0	34	0
2	4.5	1	0.5	0	480	4	6	19	1
4	12	3	4	0	830	2	10	30	3
2	1	0	0	5	570	0	4	7	2
27	26	7	3.5	155	980	8	10	30	3
5	16	4	3	5	210	10	6	44	5
0	0.5	0	0	5	40	6	0	24	0
13	10	6	0.5	50	250	45	10	76	1
9	24	7	6	55	660	8	20	86	4
4	2	1	0	5	85	15	4	31	1
4	8	2	2.5	0	270	0	10	42	1
14	20	12	1	55	190	45	6	96	1

Fast Food—McDonald's

FOOD NAME	Portion Size	Calories	
Orange Juice	12 oz	140	
Vanilla Triple Thick Shake	16 oz	550	
Breakfast			
Big Breakfast	1	730	
Biscuit	1	240	
Egg McMuffin	1	300	
Hash Browns	1 serv	140	
Hotcakes, Margarine & Syrup	1 serv	600	
Sausage Burrito	1	300	
Sausage, Egg, Cheese McGriddle	1 serv	560	
Sausage McMuffin	1	380	
Sausage McMuffin w/ Egg	1	450	
Sausage Patty	1	170	
Scrambled Eggs	2	190	
Sandwiches, Sides			
Bacon Ranch Salad Grilled Chicken	1	300	
Big Mac	1	560	
Big N' Tasty	1	470	
Caesar Salad w/ Crispy Chicken	1	300	
California Cobb Salad w/ Grilled Chicken	1	280	
Cheeseburger	1	310	
Chicken Selects Breast Strips	3 pcs	380	
Chicken McNuggets	6 pcs	250	
Double Cheeseburger	1	460	
Fillet-O-Fish	1	400	

Protein (g)	Total Fat (g)	Sat. Fat (g)	Trans Fat (g)	Chol. (mg)	Sodium (mg)	Calcium (%)	Iron (%)	Carbs (g)	Fiber (g)
2	0	0	0	0	5	2	2	33	0
13	13	8	1	50	190	45	2	96	0
27	46	14	7	465	1470	15	30	53	3
4	11	2.5	5	0	680	4	10	31	1
17	12	4.5	0	230	860	30	15	30	2
1	8	1.5	2	0	240	0	2	15	2
9	17	4	4	20	620	15	15	102	2
13	16	6	1	175	760	20	10	26	1
21	32	11	1.5	260	1300	20	15	47	1
14	22	8	0.5	45	800	25	15	31	2
20	27	10	0.5	255	950	30	20	31	2
7	15	6	0	30	310	0	2	2	0
15	12	4	0	435	200	6	10	5	0
25	13	4	1.5	55	1020	20	10	22	3
25	30	10	1.5	80	1010	25	25	47	3
24	23	8	1.5	80	790	15	25	41	3
25	13	4	1.5	55	1020	20	10	22	3
35	11	5	0	150	1120	15	10	12	4
15	12	6	1	40	740	20	15	35	1
23	20	3.5	2.5	55	930	2	4	28	0
15	15	3	1.5	35	670	2	4	15	0
25	23	11	1.5	80	1140	30	20	37	1
14	18	4	1	40	640	15	10	42	1

FOOD NAME	Portion Size	Calories
French Fries	small	250
French Fries	med	380
French Fries	large	570
Fruit & Walnut Salad	1	310
McChicken	1	370
Premium Grilled Chicken Classic Sandwich	1	420
Premium Grilled Chicken Club Sandwich	•	590
Quarterpounder w/o cheese	1	420
Quarterpounder w/ cheese	1	510
FAST FOOD—Panda Express		
BBQ Pork	5.5 oz	400
Beef w/ Broccoli	5.5 oz	150
Chicken Egg Roll	1	170
Chicken w/ Mushrooms	5.5 oz	130
Chicken w/ String Beans	5.5 oz	160
Egg Flower Soup	12 oz	88
Firecracker Beef	5.5 oz	160
Fried Shrimp	6 pcs	260
Hot and Sour Soup	12 oz	110
Kung Pao Chicken	5.5 oz	240
Kung Pao Shrimp	5.5 oz	240
Mandarin Chicken	5.5 oz	250
Mandarin Sauce	1.5 oz	70
Mixed Vegetables	5.5 oz	50
Orange Flavored Chicken	5.5 oz	500

Protein (g)	Total Fat (g)	Sat. Fat (g)	Trans Fat (g)	Chol. (mg)	Sodium (mg)	Calcium (%)	Iron (%)	Carbs (g)	Fiber (g)
2	13	2.5	3.5	0	140	2	4	30	3
4	20	4	5	0	220	2	6	47	5
6	30	6	8	0	330	2	10	70	7
5	13	2	0	5	85	15	4	44	6
15	16	3.5	1	50	810	15	15	41	1
32	9	2	0	80	1240	8	20	52	3
40	22	8	0	100	1830	30	20	64	3
24	18	7	1	70	730	15	25	40	3
29	25	12	1.5	95	1150	30	25	43	3
41	23	9	0	140	1570	na	na	15	1
11	7	1.5	0	25	510	na	na	11	4
8	8	1.5	0	25	410	na	na	17	2
8	6	1.5	0	45	520	na	na	42	3
12	8	1.5	0	25	550	na	na	10	4
2	2.2	0	0	55	895	na	na	16	0
11	8	2	0	25	670	na	na	11	4
9	13	2.5	0	60	810	na	na	26	1
5	3.5	1	0	85	1370	na	na	14	2
16	15	3	0	65	540	na	na	12	5
16	14	2	0	95	640	na	na	14	4
31	10	3	0	145	1150	na	na	8	8
1	0	0	0	0	740	na	na	17	0
3	1.5	0	0	0	370	na	na	7	3
23	27	5.5	1	100	810	na	na	42	3

FOOD NAME	Portion Size	Calories	
Steamed Rice	8 oz	380	
Sweet & Sour Pork	5.5 oz	400	
Sweet & Sour Sauce	1.5 oz	80	
Tangy Shrimp w/ Pineapple	5.5 oz	150	
Vegetable Chow Mein	8 oz	390	
Vegetable Fried Rice	8 oz	450	
Veggie Spring Roll	1	80	
FAST FOOD—Starbucks			
Beverages			
Banana Caramel Frappuccino, no whip	16 oz	410	
Caffe Latte	16 oz	260	
Caffe Vanilla Frappuccino, no whip	16 oz	340	
Cappuccino	16 oz	150	
Caramel Apple Cider, no whip	16 oz	300	
Iced Caffe Latte	16 oz	160	
Iced Caffe Mocha, whip	16 oz	350	
Iced Tazo Green Tea Latte	16 oz	250	
Tazo Black Tea Lemonade	16 oz	120	
Tazo Chai Tea Latte	16 oz	290	
Toffee Nut crème w/ whip	16 oz	450	
Vanilla Latte	16 oz	320	
Desserts/Baked Goods			
Apple Fritter	1	790	
Banana Nut Loaf	1 pc	360	
Banana Walnut Muffin	1	460	

Protein (g)	Total Fat (g)	Sat. Fat (g)	Trans Fat (g)	Chol. (mg)	Sodium (mg)	Calcium (%)	Iron (%)	Carbs (g)	Fiber (g)
9	2.5	0.5	0	30	81	na	na	81	4
13	23	4.5	0	30	360	na	na	15	1
1	0	0	0	0	135	na	na	19	0
9	5	1	0	85	550	na	na	16	2
11	12	2	0	0	1020	na	na	59	7
13	14	3	0	105	710	na	na	67	6
2	3.5	1	0	0	270	na	na	11	2
6	3.5	2.5	0	15	260	na	na	89	0
14	14	9	0	55	200	na	na	21	0
6	3.5	2	0	15	260	na	na	72	0
8	8	5	0	30	115	na	na	13	0
0	0	0	0	0	15	na	na	72	0
8	8	5	0	30	120	na	na	13	0
9	20	12	0.5	75	105	na	na	37	2
8	8	4.5	0	25	95	na	na	37	1
0	0	0	0	0	15	na	na	30	0
8	7	4.5	0	30	120	na	na	50	0
14	24	15	0	100	380	na	na	43	0
13	12	7	0	40	160	na	na	39	0
11	18	5	0	0	830	20	50	109	11
4	18	11	0	100	380	2	15	47	1
6	22	4	1	70	350	6	10	61	2

FOOD NAME	Portion Size	Calories
Black Bottom Cupcake	1	580
Black & White Cookie	1	430
Blueberry Muffin	1	420
Blueberry Scone	1	500
Bran Muffin	1	420
Butter Croissant	1	440
Chocolate Marshmallow Bar	1	410
Cinnamon Nut Croissant	1	320
Cinnamon Twist	1	320
Cranberry Muffin	1	460
Cream Cheese Danish	1	440
Crumb Cake	1	430
Fudge Brownie	1	380
Iced Lemon Pound Cake	1	500
Maple Nut Scone	1	650
Multigrain Bagel	1	360
Orange Cupcake	1	310
Sesame Bagel	1	280
Seven Layer Bar	1	600
Starbucks Espresso Brownie	1	370
Tomato & Asiago Focaccia	1	410
FAST FOOD—Subway		
6-inch Sandwiches		
Cheese Steak	1	360
Chicken & Bacon Ranch	1	530

Protein (g)	Total Fat (g)	Sat. Fat (g)	Trans Fat (g)	Chol. (mg)	Sodium (mg)	Calcium (%)	Iron (%)	Carbs (g)	Fiber (g)
6	29	8	1	80	640	4	20	72	2
4	17	3	1	50	210	2	8	68	2
5	20	4	1	65	380	2	8	55	1
6	29	18	0	100	380	6	20	56	1
8	10	2	0	45	470	10	20	58	6
7	25	16	0	70	200	0	15	47	4
5	27	12	2	60	230	6	10	61	2
5	24	12	0	50	230	4	10	22	1
4	17	1.5	5	25	280	2	8	37	1
6	23	4	1	85	410	2	10	46	1
11	34	10	7	35	750	2	0	60	1
5	25	16	8	75	140	6	15	48	3
5	15	4	2	<5	40	2	10	59	3
6	23	12	0	145	380	2	10	69	<5
7	34	13	6	40	240	6	20	80	3
12	4	0	0	0	480	4	20	72	4
2	15	5	1.5	5	230	4	6	42	1
10	0	0	0	0	460	0	20	60	4
8	37	17	2.5	10	270	15	15	63	4
4	21	13	0	84	115	4	10	72	2
15	18	5	0	0	590	30	20	48	3
24	10	4.5	0	35	1090	15	45	47	5
36	25	10	0.5	90	1400	25	25	47	5

Fast Food—Subway FOOD NAME	Portion Size	Calories	
Chicken Parmesan	1	510	
Cold Cut Combo	1	410	
Ham	1	290	
Italian BMT	1	450	
Meatball Marinara	1	560	
Oven Roasted Chicken Breast	1	330	
Roast Beef	1	290	
Spicy Italian	1	480	
Tuna	1	530	
Turkey Breast	1	280	
Turkey Breast & Ham	1	290	
Veggie Delite	1	230	
6-Inch Double Meat			
Cheese Steak	1	450	
Chipolte Southwest Cheese Steak	1	540	
Classic Tuna	1	790	
Cold Cut Combo	1	550	
Ham	1	380	
Italian BMT	1	630	
Meatball Marinara	1	960	
Oven Roasted Chicken	1	430	
Seafood Sensation	1	640	
Subway Club	1	420	
Turkey Breast	1	340	
Turkey Breast & Ham	1	360	

Protein (g)	Total Fat (g)	Sat. Fat (g)	Trans Fat (g)	Chol. (mg)	Sodium (mg)	Calcium (%)	Iron (%)	Carbs (g)	Fiber (g)
26	18	6	0	38	1410	25	25	64	5
21	17	7	0.5	60	1550	15	30	47	4
18	5	1.5	0	25	1280	6	25	47	4
23	21	8	0	55	1790	15	25	47	4
24	24	11	1	45	1610	20	40	63	7
24	5	1.5	0	25	1280	6	25	47	4
19	5	2	0	20	920	6	30	45	4
21	25	9	0	55	1670	6	25	46	4
22	31	7	0.5	45	1030	10	30	45	4
18	4.5	1.5	0	20	1020	6	25	46	4
20	5	1.5	0	25	1230	6	25	47	4
9	3	1	0	0	520	6	25	44	4
37	14	6	0	60	1470	15	60	50	6
37	24	7	0	70	1680	15	60	51	7
32	55	11	1	80	1340	10	30	45	4
31	28	10	1	110	2380	20	35	49	4
28	7	2.5	0	50	2180	6	30	57	4
34	35	14	0	100	2890	15	30	49	4
37	42	18	2	85	2490	25	50	68	4
39	8	2	0	90	1520	6	25	50	4
20	38	8.0	1	40	1580	20	25	58	5
39	8	3.5	0	65	2100	6	40	50	4
28	6	1.5	0	40	1520	6	25	48	4
31	7	2	0	50	1950	6	30	50	4

Fast Food—Subway FOOD NAME	Portion Size	Calories	
Turkey Breast, Ham & Bacon melt	1	500	
Breakfast Sandwiches & Wraps			
Cheese Sandwich	1	310	
Cheese Wrap, 1	1	220	
Chipolte Steak & Cheese Sandwich	1	470	
Chipolte Steak & Cheese Wrap	1	430	
Double Bacon & Cheese Sandwich	1	500	
Double Bacon & Cheese Wrap	1	420	
Honey Mustard Ham & Egg Sandwich	1	310	
Honey Mustard Ham & Egg Wrap	1	230	
Western w/ Cheese sandwich	1	400	
Western w/ Cheese Wrap	1	310	
Deli-style Sandwiches			
Ham	1	210	
Roast beef	1	220	
Turkey Breast	1	210	
Tuna w/ Cheese	1	350	
Desserts & Beverages			
Apple Pie	1	245	
Berry Lishus	small	110	
Berry Lishus w/ Banana	small	140	
Chocolate Chip Cookie	1	210	
Chocolate Chunk Cookie	1	220	
Double Chocolate Chip Cookie	1	210	
Fruit Roll-up	1	50	

Protein (g)	Total Fat (g)	Sat. Fat (g)	Trans Fat (g)	Chol. (mg)	Sodium (mg)	Calcium (%)	Iron (%)	Carbs (g)	Fiber (g)
40	17	8	0	82	2520	15	30	51	4
19	9	3.5	0	15	740	15	20	43	3
24	10	3.5	0	15	1040	20	10	16	8
28	25	9	0.5	50	1200	25	35	38	4
36	27	8	0	50	1600	30	25	19	9
31	23	12	0.5	60	1400	30	25	45	4
37	25	11	0.5	60	1720	35	10	18	8
20	5	1.5	0	15	1150	6	25	50	3
26	7	1	0	15	1480	10	10	23	8
27	14	7	0	40	1210	25	25	46	4
32	16	6	0	40	1540	30	10	19	8
11	18	5	0.5	10	770	8	25	36	3
13	4.5	2	0	15	660	8	25	35	3
13	3.5	1.5	0	15	730	10	25	36	3
14	18	5	0.5	30	750	10	25	35	3
0	10	2	na	0	290	0	3	37	1
1	0	0	0	0	30	0	10	28	1
2	0	0	0	0	30	0	10	35	2
2	10	4	1	15	160	0	6	30	1
2	10	3.5	2.5	10	105	0	6	30	1
2	10	4	1	15	170	0	6	30	1
0	1	0	0	0	55	0	0	12	0

FOOD NAME	Portion Size	Calories	
M&M's Cookie	1	210	
Oatmeal Raisin Cookie	1	200	
Peanut Butter Cookie	1	220	
Pineapple Delight Beverage	small	130	
Pineapple Delight w/ Banana	small	160	
Sugar Cookie	1	230	
Sunrise Refresher Beverage	small	120	
White Chip Macadamia Nut Cookie	1	220	
Soups			
Brown & Wild Rice w/ Chicken	10 oz	230	
Chicken & Dumpling	10 oz	140	
Cream of Broccoli	10 oz	140	
Cream of Potato w/ Bacon	10 oz	220	
Golden Broccoli & Cheese	10 oz	180	
Minestrone	10 oz	90	
New England Style Clam Chowder	10 oz	150	
Roasted Chicken Noodle	10 oz	90	
Spanish Style Chicken w/ Rice	10 oz	110	
Tomato Garden Vegetable w/ Rotini	10 oz	90	
Vegetable Beef	10 oz	100	
Wraps			
Chicken & Bacon Ranch w/ Cheese	1	440	
Turkey Breast	1	190	
Turkey Breast & Bacon Melt	1	380	
Tuna w/ Cheese	1	440	

Protein (g)	Total Fat (g)	Sat. Fat (g)	Trans Fat (g)	Chol. (mg)	Sodium (mg)	Calcium (%)	Iron (%)	Carbs (g)	Fiber (g)
2	10	3.5	2.5	15	105	0	6	30	1
3	8	2.5	2.5	15	170	0	6	30	2
4	12	4	1	10	200	0	6	26	1
1	0	0	0	0	25	0	0	33	1
1	0	0	0	0	25	0	0	40	2
2	12	3.5	3.5	15	135	0	6	28	0
1	0	0	0	0	20	2	0	29	1
2	11	3.5	1	15	160	0	6	28	1
6	11	3.5	0	50	1170	15	2	26	1
7	3.5	1.5	0	5	1230	4	6	20	2
8	5	2	0	10	060	15	2	18	4
5	10	4	0	15	980	10	2	28	5
5	11	5	0	25	990	8	2	16	4
4	10	1	0	<5	910	4	4	17	3
5	5	1.5	0	10	1400	8	4	20	2
6	2	0.5	0	20	1130	2	2	12	1
6	2.5	1	0	5	980	2	2	16	1
3	0.5	0	0	40	1040	6	6	20	3
5	1.5	0.5	0	10	1060	2	2	17	3
41	27	10	0.5	90	1670	30	15	18	9
24	6	1	0	20	1290	10	15	18	9
31	24	7	0	50	1780	20	15	20	9
27	32	6	0.5	45	1310	15	15	16	9

Fast Food—Taco Bell FOOD NAME	Portion Size	Calories	
FAST FOOD—Taco Bell			
Burritos			
Bean Burrito	1	370	
Burrito Supreme, Beef	1	440	
Burrito Supreme, Chicken	1	410	
Burrito Supreme, Steak	1	420	
Chili Cheese Burrito	1	390	
Grilled Stuft Burrito, Beef	1	720	
Grilled Stuft Burrito, Chicken	1	670	
Grilled Stuft Burrito, Steak	1	680	
One-half lb Beef Combo Burrito	1	470	
One-half lb Beef & Potato Burrito	1	540	
One-half lb Cheesy Bean & Rice Burrito	1	490	
Seven-Layer Burrito	1	530	
Spicy Chicken Burrito	1	420	
Chalupas			
Nacho Cheese, Beef	1	380	
Nacho Cheese, Chicken	1	350	
Nacho Cheese, Steak	1	360	
Supreme, Beef	1	400	
Supreme, Chicken	1	370	
Supreme, Steak	1	370	
Gorditas			
Baja, Beef, fresco	1	250	
Baja, Chicken, regular	1	290	

Protein (g)	Total Fat (g)	Sat. Fat (g)	Trans Fat (g)	Chol. (mg)	Sodium (mg)	Calcium (%)	Iron (%)	Carbs (g)	Fiber (g)
14	10	3.5	2	10	1200	20	15	55	8
17	18	8	2	40	1330	20	15	52	5
21	14	6	2	45	1270	20	15	50	5
19	16	7	2	35	1260	20	15	50	6
16	18	9	1.5	40	1080	30	10	40	3
27	32	11	3	55	2140	35	25	80	7
35	25	7	2.5	70	2010	30	20	77	7
31	27	8	3	55	1990	30	25	77	7
22	19	7	2	45	1620	20	20	52	5
15	25	8	3.5	30	1000	20	20	66	4
13	21	6	3	15	1430	25	15	61	6
18	21	8	2.5	25	1400	30	20	68	9
14	19	4	1.5	30	1220	15	15	51	4
12	22	5	3	20	760	10	15	33	2
16	18	4	3	25	700	10	10	31	2
14	20	4.5	3	20	690	10	15	31	2
13	24	8	2.5	35	620	15	15	31	2
17	21	7	2	45	550	15	10	29	2
15	22	7	2	35	550	15	15	29	2
12	9	3	0	20	580	6	15	30	2
17	12	5	0	45	530	10	10	28	2

Fast Food—Taco Bell FOOD NAME	Portion Size	Calories	
Baja, Steak, regular	1	320	
Supreme, Beef, fresco	1	230	
Supreme, Beef, regular	1	350	
Supreme, Chicken, fresco	1	230	
Supreme, Chicken, regular	1	290	
Supreme, Steak, fresco	1	230	
Supreme, Steak, regular	1	290	
Taco Bell			
Chicken Ranchero Taco, fresco	1	170	
Chicken Ranchero Taco, regular	1	270	
Double Decker Taco	1	340	
Grande Soft Taco	1	450	
Grilled Steak Soft Taco, fresco	1	170	
Grilled Steak Soft Taco, regular	1	280	
Soft Taco, Beef, fresco	1	190	
Soft Taco, Beef, regular	1	210	
Taco, fresco style	1	150	
Taco, regular style	1	170	
Miscellaneous			
Cheese Quesadilla	1	490	
Cheesy Fiesta Potatoes	1 scrv	290	
Chicken Quesadilla	1	540	
Cinnamon Twists	1	160	
Crunchwrap Supreme	1	560	
Enchirito, Beef	1	380	

Protein (g)	Total Fat (g)	Sat. Fat (g)	Trans Fat (g)	Chol. (mg)	Sodium (mg)	Calcium (%)	Iron (%)	Carbs (g)	Fiber (g)
15	16	4	0	30	680	10	10	29	2
13	7	1.5	0	15	510	6	10	28	2
13	19	5	0.5	30	760	15	15	31	2
15	6	1	0	25	510	6	10	28	2
17	12	5	0	45	530	10	10	28	2
13	7	1.5	0	15	510	6	10	28	2
16	13	6	0.5	35	520	10	15	28	2
12	4	1	0.5	25	560	8	6	20	2
14	14	4	0.5	35	710	10	6	21	2
14	14	5	1.5	25	810	15	10	39	5
19	21	8	2.5	45	1410	20	15	44	2
12	4	1	0.5	15	560	8	8	21	2
12	17	4.5	1	30	650	10	8	21	1
9	8	2.5	0.5	20	630	8	8	22	2
10	10	4	1	25	620	10	8	21	1
7	7	2.5	0.5	20	360	2	6	14	2
8	10	4	0.5	25	350	6	6	13	1
19	28	13	2	55	1150	50	8	39	3
4	18	6	3	15	790	6	6	28	2
28	30	13	2	80	1380	50	10	40	3
1	5	1	1	0	220	0	0	27	<1
17	24	9	3.5	35	1350	25	20	70	4
19	18	9	1.5	45	1430	25	10	35	5

Fast Food—Taco Bell – Fast Food—Wendy's FOOD NAME	Portion Size	Calories	
Enchirito, Chicken	1	350	
Enchirito, Steak	1	540	
Express Taco Salad	1	630	
Fiesta Taco Salad	1	860	
Fiesta Taco Salad, no shell	1	490	
Mexican Pizza	1	540	
Mexican Rice	1 serv	200	
Nachos, BellGrande	1	790	
Nachos, Supreme	1	460	
SW Steak Border Bowl	1	690	
Tostada	1	250	
Zesty Chicken Border Bowl	1	730	
FAST FOOD—Wendy's			
Biggie French Fries	5.6 oz	490	
Blackforest Ham & swiss frescata	1	480	
Cheeseburger, Jr.	1	320	
Chicken BLT	1	340	
Chili, large	large	330	
Fix 'n mix frosty	med	170	
Frosty	med	430	
Ham & Cheese Sandwich, Kids	1	240	
Hamburger, Jr.	1	280	
Homestyle Chicken Fillet Sandwich	1	540	
Homestyle Chicken Strips	3 strips	410	
Low-fat Strawberry Flavored Yogurt	1	140	

Protein (g)	Total Fat (g)	Sat. Fat (g)	Trans Fat (g)	Chol. (mg)	Sodium (mg)	Calcium (%)	Iron (%)	Carbs (g)	Fiber (g)
23	14	7	1.5	55	1360	25	10	33	5
26	31	14	2	70	1370	50	15	40	3
26	34	12	3.5	65	1390	25	20	58	10
31	46	14	5	65	1800	40	30	82	12
24	25	11	2	65	1350	25	20	43	10
20	31	10	3.5	45	1040	35	15	47	5
6	9	3.5	0.5	15	850	10	8	26	2
19	44	12	7	35	1300	15	15	79	10
13	26	8	3.5	30	810	10	10	42	5
30	28	8	2.5	55	2330	20	30	79	10
11	10	4	1.5	15	710	15	8	29	7
23	40	8	2.5	45	1810	15	20	69	10
5	24	4	6	0	480	2	8	64	6
28	20	6	0	65	1490	25	20	50	4
17	13	6	0.5	40	820	10	20	34	1
34	18	9	0	105	840	30	10	12	4
25	9	3.5	0.5	55	1170	10	20	35	8
4	4	2.5	0	20	80	15	8	29	0
10	11	7	0	45	200	40	20	74	0
14	6	3	0	30	890	10	20	32	1
15	9	3.5	0.5	30	600	2	20	34	1
29	22	4	1.5	55	1350	4	20	57	2
28	18	3.5	3	60	1470	2	6	33	0
6	1.5	1	0	5	85	20	2	27	0

FOOD NAME	Portion Size	Calories	
Mandarin Chicken Salad	1	170	
Nuggets	10 pcs	440	
Roasted Turkey & Basil Pesto Frescata	1	420	
Side Salad	1	35	
Southwest Taco Salad	1	440	
Spicy Chicken Fillet Sandwich	1	510	
Ultimate Chicken Grill Sandwich	1	360	
FIGS			
Canned, solids & liquid	1 c	131	
Fresh, large	2.5"	47	
Stewed	1 c	277	
Sun-Maid, Mission & Calimyrna	4	120	
FILBERTS, dry roasted, no salt	1 oz	182	
FLOUNDER, baked	3 oz	99	
Mrs. Paul's fillets	1	150	
FLOUR			
Barley	1 c	511	
Corn, whole grain, yellow	1 c	422	
Cornmeal, self-rising, enriched	1 c	592	
Gold Medal Better for Bread	¼ c	100	
Gold Medal unbleached, all-purpose	¼ c	100	
Gold Medal whole wheat	¼ c	100	
Rice, brown	1 c	574	
Rye, dark	1 c	415	
FRANKFURTERS			

Protein (g)	Total Fat (g)	Sat. Fat (g)	Trans Fat (g)	Chol. (mg)	Sodium (mg)	Calcium (%)	Iron (%)	Carbs (g)	Fiber (g)
23	2	0.5	0	60	480	6	10	18	3
21	29	6	3.5	70	970	2	6	25	0
21	16	3	0	40	1530	6	20	50	4
1	0	0	0	0	25	4	4	8	2
30	22	12	1	80	1100	45	20	32	9
29	10	3.5	1.5	55	1480	4	15	57	2
31	7	1.5	0	75	1100	4	15	44	2
1	0	0	0	0	2	7	4	35	5
0	0	0	0	0	1	2	1	12	2
4	1	0	0	0	10	18	13	71	11
0	0	0	0	0	0	6	8	28	0
4	18	1	0	0	0	3	7	5	3
21	1	0	0	58	89	2	2	0	0
8	7	3.5	0	25	290	0	2	12	1
16	2	0	0	0	6	5	22	110	15
8	5	1	0	0	6	1	15	90	16
14	5	1	0	0	2243	51	47	125	11
3	0	0	0	0	0	0	6	22	<1
3	0	0	0	0	0	0	6	22	<1
4	0.5	0	0	0	0	0	2	21	3
11	4	1	0	0	13	2	17	121	7
18	3	0	0	0	1	7	46	88	29

Frankfurters – Frankfurter Substitutes

FOOD NAME	Portion Size	Calories	
Ballpark			
Beef Franks	1	180	
Bun Size Smoked White Turkey	1	45	
Fat-free Franks	1	40	
Grillmaster Deli Style	1	250	
Grillmaster Hearty Beef	1	250	
Lite Beef	1	100	
Hebrew National			
97% f-f Beef	1	45	
¼-lb Dinner Frank	1	350	
Beef Frank	1	150	
Cocktail Franks	5 links	180	
Frank in a Blanket	5 links	290	
Oscar Mayer			
Beef Bun-Length	1	180	
Beef Franks	1	140	
Beef Jumbo	1	180	
Beef Light	1	90	
Beef XXL Deli Style	1	230	
Cheese Dogs	1	140	
Turkey Franks	1	100	
Wieners, f-f	1	40	
Wieners, Jumbo	1	180	
XXL Hot & Spicy	1	210	
FRANKFURTER SUBSTITUTES			

Protein (g)	Total Fat (g)	Sat. Fat (g)	Trans Fat (g)	Chol. (mg)	Sodium (mg)	Calcium (%)	Iron (%)	Carbs (g)	Fiber (g)
6	16	7	0	35	550	0	5	3	0
6	0	0	0	10	420	0	2	5	0
5	0	0	0	10	420	0	2	4	0
8	23	9	0	50	830	0	6	3	0
9	23	9	0	50	780	0	6	3	0
6	7	3	0	25	450	0	4	3	0
6	1.5	1	0	15	400	0	6	3	0
13	32	15	0	70	990	0	8	1	0
6	14	6	0	30	370	0	4	1	0
7	16	7	0	40	450	0	4	1	0
9	24	10	0	40	690	0	8	8	1
6	17	7	1	35	580	0	4	2	0
5	13	6	1	30	460	0	2	1	0
6	17	7	1	35	580	0	4	2	0
5	6	6	0	20	500	0	4	2	0
9	22	9	1.5	50	740	0	8	1	0
5	13	4	0	35	540	6	2	1	0
5	8	2.5	0	30	510	2	4	2	0
6	0	0	0	15	490	0	2	3	0
6	17	7	1	35	580	0	4	2	0
10	19	8	0	45	780	0	6	3	0

Frankfurter Substitutes – Frosting	Portion Size	Calories	
FOOD NAME			
Morningstar Corn Dog	1	150	
Morningstar Veggie Dog	1	80	
Worthington Corn Dog	1	150	
Worthington Little Links	2	90	
Worthington Low-fat Big Franks	1	80	
Yves, Hot & Spicy Chili Veggie	1	74	
Yves, Tofu Dog	1	47	
Yves, Veggie Dog	1	56	
FRENCH TOAST			
Aunt Jemima Cinnamon French Toast	2 slices	240	
Murry's French Toast Sticks	5	300	
Pillsbury French Toast Sticks, Cinnamon	6	350	
Pillsbury French Toast Sticks, Homestyle	6	310	
FROSTING			
Betty Crocker			
Homestyle Fluffy White, f-f, prep	6 Tbs	100	
Rich & Creamy Butter Cream	2 Tbs	150	
Rich & Creamy Caramel	2 Tbs	150	
Rich & Creamy Cherry	2 Tbs	150	
Rich & Creamy Chocolate	2 Tbs	140	
Rich & Creamy Coconut Pecan	2 Tbs	140	
Rich & Creamy Cream Cheese	2 Tbs	150	
Rich & Creamy Lemon	2 Tbs	150	
Rich & Creamy Rainbow Chip	2 Tbs	140	

Protein (g)	Total Fat (g)	Sat. Fat (g)	Trans Fat (g)	Chol. (mg)	Sodium (mg)	Calcium (%)	Iron (%)	Carbs (g)	Fiber (g)
7	4	0.5	0	0	500	0	6	22	3
11	0.5	0	0	0	580	0	4	6	1
7	4	0.5	0	0	500	0	6	22	3
8	5	0.5	0	0	250	0	2	3	2
12	2.5	0.5	0	0	240	0	4	3	2
13	1	0	0	0	395	0	19	3	0
9	0.5	0	0	0	241	0	16	2	0
11	0	0	0	0	399	0	16	1	0
8	6	1.5	0	70	340	10	15	39	2
5	11	2	0	20	400	4	10	48	1
4	6	2	1.5	10	640	6	20	69	1
4	6	2	1.5	10	650	2	20	68	1
<1	0	0	0	0	55	0	0	24	0
0	7	2	2.5	0	80	0	0	20	0
0	7	2	2.5	0	85	0	0	20	0
0	7	2	2.5	0	80	0	0	21	0
0	7	2	2.5	0	100	0	4	18	<1
0	7	3	1.5	0	55	0	0	18	<1
0	7	2	2.5	0	80	0	0	20	0
0	8	3	2.5	0	85	0	0	20	0
0	5	2	1.5	0	70	0	0	23	0

Frosting – Frozen Breakfast (also see "French Toast" and "Pancakes") FOOD NAME	Portion Size	Calories	
Rich & Creamy Triple Chocolate			
Fudge Chip	2 Tbs	140	
Rich & Creamy Vanilla	2 Tbs	150	
Whipped Butter Cream	2 Tbs	110	
Whipped Chocolate	2 Tbs	100	
Whipped Chocolate Mousse	2 Tbs	90	
Whipped Cream Cheese	2 Tbs	110	
Whipped Lemon	2 Tbs	110	
Whipped Milk Chocolate	2 Tbs	100	
Whipped Vanilla	2 Tbs	110	
Whipped Whipped Cream	2 Tbs	100	
FROZEN BREAKFAST (also see "French Toast" and "Pancakes")			
Amy's Kitchen, Breakfast Burrito	1	250	
Jimmy Dean Omelet, Three Cheese	1	270	
Jimmy Dean Omelet, Ham & Cheese	1	280	
Jimmy Dean Omelet, Sausage & Cheese	1	270	
Jimmy Dean Omelet, Western Style	1	270	
Jimmy Dean Wrap, Sausage, Egg, Cheese	1	320	
Morningstar Farms Breakfast Sandwich			
w/ Cheese	1	250	
Pillsbury Toaster Scrambles,			
Bacon & Sausage	1	180	
Pillsbury Toaster Scrambles, Cheese,			
Egg, Bacon	1	180	

Protein (g)	Total Fat (g)	Sat. Fat (g)	Trans Fat (g)	Chol. (mg)	Sodium (mg)	Calcium (%)	Iron (%)	Carbs (g)	Fiber (g)
1	5	1.5	1.5	0	90	0	4	22	<1
0	7	2	2.5	0	80	0	0	21	0
0	5	1.5	1.5	0	25	0	0	15	0
<1	5	1.5	1	0	55	0	4	14	0
0	4.5	1.5	1	0	55	0	4	14	1
0	5	1.5	1.5	0	45	0	0	15	0
0	5	1.5	1.5	0	25	0	0	15	0
0	4.5	1.5	1	0	50	0	4	14	0
0	5	1.5	1.5	0	25	0	0	15	0
0	5	1.5	1.5	0	25	0	0	15	0
9	7	0.5	0	0	540	6	20	38	5
15	21	10	0	385	830	25	8	5	1
15	17	7	0	325	770	15	8	5	0
15	22	8	0	295	570	15	8	4	0
13	14	4.5	0	245	590	10	8	5	1
14	17	7	0.5	185	850	20	10	25	1
28	3	0.5	0	10	1000	30	40	35	5
4	12	3	1.5	20	360	0	4	15	0
4	12	3	1.5	25	370	0	4	15	0

Frozen Breakfast – Frozen Dinners & Entrées FOOD NAME	Portion Size	Calories	
Pillsbury Toaster Scrambles, Cheese/Egg/Sausage	1	180	
South Beach Diet Breakfast Wrap, All-American	1	200	
South Beach Diet Breakfast Wrap, Denver	1	180	
South Beach Diet Breakfast Wrap, Southwest Style	1	160	
South Beach Diet Breakfast Wrap, Vegetable	1	160	
FROZEN DINNERS & ENTRÉES			
Amy's Kitchen			
Asian Noodle Stir-Fry	1 pkg	240	
Black Bean Vegetable Enchilada	1	280	
Broccoli Pot Pie	1	430	
Brown rice, Black-Eyed Peas and Veggies bowl	1	290	
Brown rice & Vegetables Bowl	1	260	
Country Vegetable Pie	1	370	
Indian Mattar Paneer	1 pkg	320	
Indian Samosa Wraps	1 wrap	260	
Indian Vegetable Korma	1 pkg	300	
Macaroni & Cheese	1 pkg	410	
Mexican Casserole Bowl	1	480	
Mexican Tamale Pie	1	150	
Nondairy Vegetable Pot Pie	1	360	

Protein (g)	Total Fat (g)	Sat. Fat (g)	Trans Fat (g)	Chol. (mg)	Sodium (mg)	Calcium (%)	Iron (%)	Carbs (g)	Fiber (g)
4	11	3	1.5	20	360	0	4	15	0
19	9	4	0	15	620	30	4	26	15
16	7	3	0	15	620	25	4	27	15
15	5	2.5	0	10	520	25	6	26	15
14	6	3	0	5	430	25	6	26	15
7	4.5	0.5	0	0	680	8	20	41	4
0	8	1	0	0	580	8	20	44	4
11	22	10	0	45	630	15	8	46	4
11	11	1.5	0	0	580	6	15	38	8
9	9	1	0	0	550	8	10	36	5
12	16	9	0	40	580	20	15	47	4
11	8	1.5	0	5	780	10	15	54	6
8	8	1	0	0	680	4	15	38	4
9	12	3.5	0	0	680	6	20	41	7
16	16	10	0	40	590	30	10	47	3
10	18	5	0	20	780	25	20	70	7
5	3	0	0	0	590	4	10	27	4
10	13	1.5	0	0	640	6	15	50	4

Frozen Dinners & Entrées FOOD NAME	Portion Size	Calories	
Pesto Tortelli Bowl	1	430	
Ravioli Bowl	1	380	
Rice Macaroni & Cheese	1 pkg	400	
Santa Fe Enchilada Bowl	1	350	
Shepherd's Pie	1	160	
Stuffed Pasta Shells Bowl	1	310	
Teriyaki Bowl	1	280	
Thai Noodle Stir-Fry	1 pkg	310	
Tofu Vegetable Lasagna	1 pkg	300	
Vegetable Pot Pie	1	420	
Whole Meals: Black Bean Enchilada	1 meal	330	
Whole Meals: Cheese Eenchilada	1 meal	350	
Whole Meals: Chili & Cornbread	1 meal	340	
Whole Meals: Country Dinner	1 meal	390	
Whole Meals: Veggie Loaf	1 meal	280	
Bertolli			
Grilled Chicken Alfredo	½ pkg	710	
Roast Chicken & Linguini	½ pkg	420	
Shrimp, Asparagus & Penne	½ pkg	480	
Birds Eye—Voila!			
Alfredo Chicken, cooked	1 c	320	
Beef Steak & Garlic Potatoes, cooked	1 c	190	
Chicken Fajita, cooked	1 c	150	
Chicken & Sausage, reduced carbs, cooked	1 c	170	

Protein (g)	Total Fat (g)	Sat. Fat (g)	Trans Fat (g)	Chol. (mg)	Sodium (mg)	Calcium (%)	Iron (%)	Carbs (g)	Fiber (g)
20	19	8	0	40	640	40	10	45	3
14	12	4.5	0	25	680	20	15	55	4
16	16	10	0	50	590	30	10	47	1
16	11	2	0	5	780	10	20	47	10
5	4	0	0	0	490	10	15	27	5
19	13	7	0	30	740	40	15	30	5
10	3.5	0	0	0	780	4	8	52	4
8	11	7	0	0	420	4	4	45	5
13	10	1.5	0	0	630	10	25	41	6
9	19	12	0	50	590	4	8	54	4
9	8	1	0	0	740	6	15	53	9
15	15	7	0	30	680	30	15	38	6
11	6	2.5	0	10	680	10	15	59	10
11	12	4	0	15	680	10	10	60	8
8	7	1	0	47	690	4	15	47	7
29	42	22	1.5	220	1210	20	8	54	4
25	17	4.5	0	75	1500	20	6	41	4
16	21	9	0	90	1300	15	8	50	4
14	17	10	0	60	480	10	10	26	2
9	7	1.5	1	15	630	4	10	22	5
10	6	1	1	25	730	2	4	13	3
14	8	2.5	0	35	620	2	2	10	4

Frozen Dinners & Entrées FOOD NAME	Portion Size	Calories
Chicken Stir-fry, cooked	1 c	160
Garden Herb Chicken, cooked	1 c	280
Garlic Chicken, cooked	1 c	240
Garlic Shrimp, cooked	1 c	220
Pesto Chicken Primavera, cooked	1 c	210
Teriyaki Beef & Vegetables, reduced carb, cooked	1 c	160
Teriyaki Chicken, cooked	1 c	250
Three Cheese Chicken, cooked	1 c	210
Gorton's		
Alfredo Fillet Meal	1	160
Alfredo Shrimp Bowl	1	250
Beer Batter Fillets	2	230
Classic Grilled Salmon	1	100
Crispy Battered Fillets	2	260
Crunchy Golden Fillets	2	240
Fish Sticks	6	250
Fried Rice Shrimp Bowl	1	350
Garlic & Herb Fish Fillets	2	230
Grilled Fillets, Caesar Parmesan	1	100
Grilled Fillets, Cajun Blackened	1	100
Grilled Fillets, Lemon Pepper	1	100
Lemon & Herb Butter Fillet	1 meal	240
Original Batter Tenders	4 oz	270
Parmesan Breaded Fillets	2	250

Protein (g)	Total Fat (g)	Sat. Fat (g)	Trans Fat (g)	Chol. (mg)	Sodium (mg)	Calcium (%)	Iron (%)	Carbs (g)	Fiber (g)
10	3	0.5	1	15	1030	4	6	22	2
14	11	5	1	36	600	10	6	30	3
11	8	2	1	30	940	4	6	21	3
9	8	2	1.5	10	510	6	4	27	2
12	7	2	1	20	590	10	6	24	2
15	4	1.5	0	25	950	2	4	15	4
12	2.5	0	0	20	980	4	4	44	2
13	8	3	0.5	30	940	15	4	21	2
19	3	1.5	0	40	990	10	2	14	5
13	5	1.5	0	75	1230	15	10	39	4
9	14	2.5	0	20	640	2	2	18	0
15	3.5	0.5	0	20	310	0	2	1	0
9	17	3	0	30	770	2	2	17	0
9	12	2.5	0	30	500	2	6	23	0
11	14	3.5	0	20	380	2	4	20	0
13	2.5	0.5	0	40	990	10	2	14	5
9	12	2	0	30	770	2	4	22	0
17	3	0.5	0	60	250	2	2	1	0
17	3	0.5	0	60	330	2	4	1	0
17	3	0.5	0	60	380	0	2	1	0
17	3.5	1	0	40	890	6	4	34	3
9	15	3	0	25	770	0	8	25	0
10	15	3	0	30	650	2	4	19	0

Frozen Dinners & Entrées	Portion Size	Calories	
FOOD NAME			
Popcorn Fish	11 pcs	280	
Popcorn Shrimp, Beer Batter	18 pcs	270	
Popcorn Shrimp, original	20 pcs	240	
Primavera Shrimp bowl	1	270	
Ranch Fillets	2	240	
Teriyaki Shrimp bowl	1	320	
Green Giant—Complete Skillet Meals			
Chicken Alfredo, prep	1¼ c	270	
Chicken & Cheesy Pasta, prep	1¼ c	270	
Chicken Lo Mein, prep	1 c	190	
Chicken Teriyaki, prep	1½ c	240	
Garlic Chicken Pasta, prep	1 c	230	
Sweet & Sour Chicken, prep	1¼ c	320	
Green Giant Create A Meal			
Spicy Teriyaki, prep	1 c	210	
Stir-Fry Lo Mein, prep	1 c	270	
Stir-Fry Sesame, prep	1 c	260	
Sweet 'n Sour, prep	1 c	280	
Szechuan, prep	1 c	190	
Teriyaki, prep	1 c	180	
Healthy Choice, Complete Selections			
Asiago Chicken Portobello	1 pkg	330	
Beef Pot Roast	1 pkg	310	
Beef Stroganoff	1 pkg	340	
Charbroiled Beef Patty	1 pkg	310	

Protein (g)	Total Fat (g)	Sat. Fat (g)	Trans Fat (g)	Chol. (mg)	Sodium (mg)	Calcium (%)	Iron (%)	Carbs (g)	Fiber (g)
10	17	4.5	0	25	800	2	6	22	0
7	16	4.5	0	80	900	2	8	24	0
8	12	3.5	0	55	630	2	6	24	0
13	6	2.5	0	35	1250	10	10	41	1
9	13	2.5	0	30	650	2	6	22	0
10	6	1	0	45	1250	15	8	57	2
16	4.5	2	0	25	740	10	10	37	3
18	6	3	0	40	950	8	15	37	3
12	2	0	0	20	740	4	10	31	3
13	1	0	0	20	780	4	10	48	3
13	6	2.5	0	30	840	6	8	33	4
14	1.5	0	0	25	550	4	15	62	3
22	7	1	0	50	850	4	8	16	3
24	7	1.5	0	50	780	4	10	28	2
27	12	2	0	60	1160	6	8	12	4
22	7	1	0	55	540	4	8	36	3
18	9	2.5	0	40	900	4	10	10	3
22	6	1	0	50	700	4	8	11	3
20	6	2.5	0	30	600	10	10	47	6
15	7	3	0	45	500	4	10	45	5
20	9	2	0	50	460	6	6	44	5
18	9	3	0	40	600	4	10	37	6

Frozen Dinners & Entrées

FOOD NAME	Portion Size	Calories
Chicken Broccoli Alfredo	1 pkg	300
Chicken Enchilada	1 pkg	310
Chicken Parmegiana	1 pkg	320
Chicken Teriyaki	1 pkg	280
Country Breaded Chicken	1 pkg	370
Creamy Garlic Shrimp	1 pkg	280
Grilled Turkey Breast	1 pkg	250
Herb Baked Fish	1 pkg	360
Honey Glazed Chicken	1 pkg	270
Lemon Pepper Fish	1 pkg	280
Oven Roasted Beef	1 pkg	280
Roasted Chicken Breast	1 pkg	290
Sesame Chicken	1 pkg	330
Stuffed Pasta Shells	1 pkg	290
Sweet & Sour Chicken	1 pkg	350
Traditional Turkey breast	1 pkg	300
Healthy Choice, Simple Selections		
Beef Teriyaki	1 pkg	310
Cheesy Rice & Chicken	1 pkg	220
Chicken Breast & Vegetables	1 pkg	270
Chicken Fettuccini Alfredo	1 pkg	210
Chicken Piccata	1 pkg	270
Chicken Rigatoni	1 pkg	250
Four Cheese Manicotti	1 pkg	270
Grilled Chicken & Mashed Potatoes	1 pkg	160

Protein (g)	Total Fat (g)	Sat. Fat (g)	Trans Fat (g)	Chol. (mg)	Sodium (mg)	Calcium (%)	Iron (%)	Carbs (g)	Fiber (g)
17	5	2	0	25	430	10	10	46	8
16	7	2.5	0	40	600	15	10	46	6
19	9	3	na	20	600	8	10	40	6
15	4	1	0	25	550	6	4	44	8
15	9	2	0	25	550	6	6	55	8
13	5	1.5	0	25	600	10	8	44	5
18	5	2	0	35	600	4	10	31	5
16	8	2	0	40	590	4	4	55	5
15	6	2	0	35	600	4	6	39	4
13	5	2	0	20	580	2	2	46	4
22	7	2.5	0	60	600	2	10	33	5
16	7	2	0	25	600	<1	10	39	10
24	8	2	0	50	600	6	10	38	5
17	6	3	0	20	350	40	10	40	7
15	9	3	0	10	600	4	8	50	6
21	4	1	0	25	550	4	10	42	6
16	7	2.5	0	40	600	2	8	44	5
15	6	2.5	0	30	600	10	4	24	5
18	7	2	0	40	550	4	8	30	6
16	5	2	0	25	570	10	10	23	5
16	5	2.5	0	35	600	2	2	39	2
14	7	2	0	25	600	4	8	30	5
12	4.5	2.5	0	15	450	15	10	44	5
11	3.5	1.5	0	25	420	4	4	18	3

Frozen Dinners & Entrées FOOD NAME	Portion Size	Calories	
Lasagna Bake	1 pkg	270	
Macaroni & Cheese	1 pkg	210	
Oriental Style Chicken	1 pkg	230	
Sirloin Beef Tips & Mushroom Sauce	1 pkg	270	
Spaghetti w/ Meat Sauce	1 pkg	220	
Lean Cuisine—Café Classics			
Beef Portobello	1 pkg	210	
Chicken w/ Almonds	1 pkg	260	
Chicken Carbonara	1 pkg	270	
Chicken Fried Rice	1 pkg	280	
Fiesta Grilled Chicken	1 pkg	250	
Garlic Beef & Broccoli	1 pkg	170	
Shrimp & Angel Hair	1 pkg	240	
Sweet & Sour Chicken	1 pkg	300	
Teriyaki Steak	1 pkg	280	
Three Cheese Chicken	1 pkg	230	
Three Cheese Stuffed Rigatoni	1 pkg	240	
Lean Cuisine—Comfort Classics			
Baked Chicken	1 pkg	240	
Baked Lemon Pepper Fish	1 pkg	230	
Beef Pot Roast	1 pkg	190	
Beef Peppercorn	1 pkg	220	
Cheese Lasagna w/ Chicken Scaloppini	1 pkg	280	
Honey Roasted Pork	1 pkg	230	
Meatloaf & Whipped Potatoes	1 pkg	250	

Protein (g)	Total Fat (g)	Sat. Fat (g)	Trans Fat (g)	Chol. (mg)	Sodium (mg)	Calcium (%)	Iron (%)	Carbs (g)	Fiber (g)
13	7	2.5	na	20	600	10	10	38	4
9	4	2	0	5	600	15	10	32	4
19	4	1	0	30	550	2	8	28	4
20	6	2	0	35	600	2	6	35	4
10	3.5	1	0	10	510	6	10	36	5
15	5	2.5	0	30	670	6	8	25	2
17	4.5	0.5	0	30	580	4	6	38	3
20	6	2	0	30	680	10	6	34	2
17	6	1	0	50	690	4	6	39	3
19	7	3	0	45	620	15	6	27	3
15	6	2	0	30	690	8	10	13	3
15	4.5	1	0	55	600	10	4	34	2
17	3	0.5	0	30	680	2	2	51	1
19	6	2	0	30	680	4	10	37	3
21	10	3	0	45	520	15	4	14	2
12	6	3	0	20	660	20	6	35	4
15	4.5	1	0	25	650	4	6	34	3
20	6	2	0	45	690	20	6	34	3
13	6	1.5	0	25	690	6	8	22	3
14	7	2.5	0	25	690	10	8	25	3
19	2	0	0	30	580	15	8	34	5
18	9	3.5	0	50	580	6	8	18	5
20	7	2.5	0	40	580	10	15	27	3

Frozen Dinners & Entrées		
FOOD NAME	Portion Size	Calories
Roast Turkey & Vegetables	1 pkg	150
Salisbury Steak	1 pkg	280
Southern Beef Tips	1 pkg	250
Lean Cuisine—Dinnertime Selects		
Chicken Florentine	1 pkg	390
Chicken Portobello	1 pkg	380
Grilled Chicken & Penne Pasta	1 pkg	330
Jumbo Rigatoni w/ Meatballs	1 pkg	390
Lemon Garlic Shrimp	1 pkg	280
Orange Peel Chicken	1 pkg	400
Lean Cuisine—One Dish Favorites		
Asian Style Pot Stickers	1 pkg	320
Cheese Ravioli	1 pkg	250
Chicken Chow Mein w/ Rice	1 pkg	190
Chicken Enchilada Suiza	1 pkg	270
Four Cheese Cannelloni	1 pkg	240
Macaroni & Beef	1 pkg	250
Mandarin Chicken	1 pkg	240
Santa Fe Style Rice & Beans	1 pkg	290
Stuffed Cabbage w/ Whipped Potatoes	1 pkg	200
Swedish Meatballs w/ Pasta	1 pkg	280
Three Bean Chili w/ Rice	1 pkg	270
Vegetable Eggroll	1 pkg	310
Lean Cuisine—Skillets		
Asian Style Chicken & Vegetables	1 pkg	160

Protein (g)	Total Fat (g)	Sat. Fat (g)	Trans Fat (g)	Chol. (mg)	Sodium (mg)	Calcium (%)	Iron (%)	Carbs (g)	Fiber (g)
15	5	1	0	25	650	6	4	12	3
24	9	4.5	0	50	610	10	15	25	3
15	5	2	0	25	630	4	8	36	3
28	8	3.5	0	45	840	35	10	52	6
25	7	2	0	40	650	4	8	54	3
20	4.5	1.5	0	40	580	10	8	52	6
23	8	2.5	0	35	830	15	15	56	7
18	7	3.5	0	90	830	6	10	35	4
15	10	1.5	0	25	840	8	8	62	3
11	6	2	0	20	610	4	10	55	3
11	6	3.5	0	40	600	15	8	36	3
13	2.5	0.5	0	25	650	4	4	29	2
10	4.5	2	0	20	510	15	4	47	3
17	7	3.5	0	25	670	25	4	26	3
16	5	2	0	15	550	8	10	36	4
14	4	1	0	25	610	2	4	36	2
10	6	2.5	0	15	590	20	10	49	5
11	6	1.5	0	15	690	8	8	25	4
22	7	3	0	50	630	10	10	32	2
9	.7	2	0	10	620	15	15	42	8
7	5	1	0	5	640	4	6	60	3
12	2.5	0.5	0	20	610	2	6	22	2

Frozen Dinners & Entrées FOOD NAME	Portion Size	Calories	
Chicken Alfredo	1 pkg	190	
Chicken Primavera	1 pkg	180	
Chicken Teriyaki	1 pkg	230	
Garlic Chicken	1 pkg	240	
Herb Chicken	1 pkg	160	
Roasted Turkey	1 pkg	130	
Three Cheese Chicken	1 pkg	200	
Lean Cuisine—Spa Cuisine			
Chicken Mediterranean	1 pkg	220	
Chicken in Peanut Sauce	1 pkg	280	
Oven Roasted Beef Burgundy	1 pkg	300	
Pork w/ Cherry Sauce	1 pkg	260	
Rosemary Chicken	1 pkg	220	
Salmon w/ Basil	1 pkg	230	
Salmon w/ Lemon Dill Sauce	1 pkg	240	
On-Cor			
Chicken & Dumplings	1 c	170	
Chicken Parmesan	1 patty	260	
Macaroni & Cheese	1 c	170	
Salisbury Steak & Gravy	1 patty	200	
Stuffed Green Pepper	1 pc	230	
Stouffer's—Corner Bistro			
Chicken Carbonara	1 pkg	530	
Garlic Chicken Pasta	1 pkg	340	
Grilled Chicken Rosemary	1pkg	420	

Protein (g)	Total Fat (g)	Sat. Fat (g)	Trans Fat (g)	Chol. (mg)	Sodium (mg)	Calcium (%)	Iron (%)	Carbs (g)	Fiber (g)
13	4.5	2	0	25	490	10	6	25	3
12	2.5	0.5	0	20	430	2	8	28	1
12	2	1	0	25	610	4	4	40	4
12	4	2	0	25	610	2	4	40	3
11	3.5	1	0	20	560	10	6	22	3
7	1.5	0.5	0	15	450	2	4	23	3
13	5	2	0	20	420	15	8	25	3
16	4	0.5	0	20	590	10	10	30	3
22	8	1.5	0	25	680	10	10	30	3
17	7	3	0	35	640	10	10	43	3
15	4	1.5	0	30	520	4	8	41	4
17	4	2	0	35	610	6	6	29	3
19	6	2	0	25	660	15	10	25	5
16	6	2.5	0	30	690	4	8	30	4
8	8	2.5	0.5	25	610	8	4	18	1
9	14	4	0.3	20	850	4	8	18	3
8	3	2	0	10	1000	15	4	24	1
10	13	6	1	30	790	4	8	8	1
7	14	6	1	35	1030	4	10	20	1
33	22	12	na	110	1380	25	10	50	4
25	8	2	0	40	1000	15	15	43	5
25	17	5	0	60	1060	20	10	42	4

Frozen Dinners & Entrées

FOOD NAME	Portion Size	Calories	
Philly Style Steak & Cheese Panini	1 pkg	340	
Seafood Scampi	1 pkg	410	
Southwestern Style Chicken Panini	1 pkg	360	
Stouffer's—Dinners			
Chicken Fettuccini	1 pkg	620	
Meatloaf	1 pkg	560	
Roast Turkey Breast	1 pkg	390	
Slow Roast Beef	1 pkg	320	
Stouffer's—Entrées & Grilled Entrees			
Chicken a la King	1 pkg	410	
Fried Chicken Breast	1 pkg	360	
Grilled Chicken Teriyaki	1 pkg	300	
Grilled Herb Chicken	1 pkg	250	
Grilled Lemon Pepper Chicken	1 pkg	250	
Stouffer's—Skillets			
Chicken Alfredo	½ pkg	410	
Chicken & Pasta	½ pkg	340	
Homestyle Beef	½ pkg	300	
Teriyaki Chicken	½ pkg	310	
Weight Watchers—Smart Ones			
Angel Hair Marinara	1 pkg	230	
Broccoli & Cheddar Roasted Potatoes	1 pkg	220	
Chicken Carbonara	1 pkg	250	
Chicken Fettucini	1 pkg	340	
Chicken Mirabella	1 pkg	180	

Protein (g)	Total Fat (g)	Sat. Fat (g)	Trans Fat (g)	Chol. (mg)	Sodium (mg)	Calcium (%)	Iron (%)	Carbs (g)	Fiber (g)
20	16	6	0	40	680	20	15	33	3
21	11	5	0	80	999	8	10	57	6
20	16	7	0	45	920	25	15	31	3
33	24	6	0	50	1360	25	8	69	7
34	29	12	1.5	110	1180	10	20	40	8
21	13	3.5	0	40	1290	8	10	48	6
19	15	4.5	0	40	1220	6	10	27	5
18	14	4	0	50	1030	15	10	53	2
20	18	4.5	0	45	880	2	6	30	2
21	3.5	1	0	40	880	6	10	45	3
19	6	1	0	35	740	4	6	29	3
20	7	2	0	45	670	4	10	27	5
28	11	5	0	60	1080	25	15	49	2
28	7	2	0	40	410	15	10	42	6
19	11	3	0	40	1390	4	15	32	6
23	4.5	1	0	50	1130	4	6	44	6
12	1.5	0.5	0	25	340	2	4	41	2
9	6	3	0	15	480	15	6	34	5
20	4.5	1.5	0	40	660	10	8	32	2
26	8	3.5	0.5	50	620	20	15	42	4
12	2	0.5	0	15	550	6	8	33	3

FOOD NAME	Portion Size	Calories	
Chicken Parmesan	1 pkg	290	
Creamy Rigatoni w/ Broccoli & Chicken	1 pkg	290	
Dragon Shrimp Lo Mein	1 pkg	240	
Fajita Chicken Supreme	1 pkg	260	
Golden Baked Garlic Chicken	1 pkg	270	
Honey Dijon Chicken	1 pkg	220	
Lasagna Florentine	1 pkg	290	
Meatloaf w/ Gravy	1 pkg	260	
Penne Pollo	1 pkg	280	
Peppersteak	1 pkg	250	
Radiatore Romano	1 pkg	290	
Ravioli Florentine	1 pkg	250	
Roast Beef w/ Gravy	1 pkg	210	
Salisbury Steak	1 pkg	260	
Santa Fe Style Rice and Beans	1 pkg	310	
Shrimp Marinara	1 pkg	180	
Slow Roasted Turkey Breast	1 pkg	210	
Southwest Style Adobe Chicken	1 pkg	310	
Swedish Meatballs	1 pkg	270	
Thai Chicken & Rice Noodles	1 pkg	260	
Three Cheese Ziti Marinara	1 pkg	290	
Tuna noodle gratin	1 pkg	250	
FROZEN SANDWICHES/POCKETS			
Amy's Kitchen			
Broccoli & Cheese in a Pocket Sandwich	1	270	

Protein (g)	Total Fat (g)	Sat. Fat (g)	Trans Fat (g)	Chol. (mg)	Sodium (mg)	Calcium (%)	Iron (%)	Carbs (g)	Fiber (g)
26	5	1.5	0	40	630	20	10	35	4
20	8	3	0	55	690	20	10	33	2
14	4	1	0	75	690	4	20	36	3
17	7	3	0	40	600	10	6	32	4
17	5	1	0	25	670	2	4	42	2
11	3.5	0.5	0	30	460	4	4	38	2
15	9	5	0	30	580	30	10	35	4
24	8	2.5	0	35	760	10	20	22	5
21	6	2.5	0	45	510	15	15	39	3
15	4.5	1.5	0	25	710	2	10	36	3
13	7	3	0	15	490	20	10	43	4
11	5	2	0	30	720	15	10	40	4
14	9	3	0	45	550	2	4	19	2
23	7	3	0	40	820	10	15	26	3
10	7	3	0	15	660	20	6	51	4
9	1.5	0	0	20	750	8	10	31	4
18	7	2	0	45	770	2	4	18	2
14	10	3	0	75	690	4	20	36	3
20	5	2	0	30	730	15	15	35	3
14	4	0.5	0	25	570	4	4	43	2
12	7	2.5	0	10	530	15	10	44	4
14	4.5	1.5	0	45	780	15	10	37	2
8	10	4	0	15	560	20	10	37	3

Frozen Sandwiches/Pockets FOOD NAME	Portion Size	Calories	
Cheese Pizza in a Pocket Sandwich	1	300	
Roasted Vegetable in a Pocket Sandwich	1	230	
Soy Cheese Pizza in a Pocket Sandwich	1	260	
Spinach Feta in a Pocket Sandwich	1	260	
Spinach Pizza in a Pocket Sandwich	1	280	
Tofu Scramble in a Pocket Sandwich	1	180	
Vegetable Pie in a Pocket Sandwich	1	300	
Croissant Pockets			
Chicken Alfredo	1	320	
Egg, Sausage, Cheese	1	360	
Ham & Cheese	1	340	
Pepperoni Pizza	1	390	
Philly Cheese Steak	1	360	
Hot Pockets			
Three Cheese & Chicken Quesadilla	1	320	
Four Cheese Pizza	1	380	
Four Meat & Four Cheese	1	300	
Beef Taco	1	320	
Cheeseburger	1	340	
Chicken Fajita	1	290	
Ham & Cheese	1	310	
Italian Three Meat Pizza	1	350	
Meatballs & Mozzarella	1	330	
Sausage Pizza	1	360	
Supreme Pizza	1	380	

Protein (g)	Total Fat (g)	Sat. Fat (g)	Trans Fat (g)	Chol. (mg)	Sodium (mg)	Calcium (%)	Iron (%)	Carbs (g)	Fiber (g)
14	9	3.5	0	15	450	20	15	42	4
6	8	1.5	0	0	490	2	8	45	3
12	8	0.5	0	0	540	2	15	39	1
11	9	4.5	0	20	590	25	20	34	3
13	9	4	0	15	460	20	8	37	3
11	6	0	0	0	520	0	4	23	<1
8	9	1.5	0	0	490	2	8	45	3
10	15	7	0	20	690	15	15	38	3
11	20	7	0	75	620	15	15	37	3
11	15	8	0	25	760	20	15	39	3
11	20	10	0	20	810	20	15	42	3
12	19	8	0	25	810	15	15	36	3
11	13	6	0	20	700	20	15	41	3
10	20	7	0	35	800	30	15	44	3
12	19	9	na	50	790	20	15	38	3
12	13	6	0	30	910	20	15	40	3
11	14	6	0	35	700	15	15	43	3
10	11	4	0	30	670	15	15	39	3
12	13	5	na	30	770	20	15	36	3
11	16	6	0	30	890	20	10	42	3
10	14	5	0	30	770	20	15	42	3
10	19	7	0	25	710	20	15	40	3
10	20	8	0	30	630	20	15	41	3

Frozen Sandwiches/Pockets – Gelatin FOOD NAME	Portion Size	Calories	
Lean Pockets			
Cheeseburger	1	280	
Chicken Parmesan	1	280	
Five Cheese Pizza	1	390	
Meatball & Mozzarella	1	330	
Philly Steak & Cheese	1	280	
Sausage, Egg & Cheese	1	140	
Sausage & Pepperoni	1	280	
Turkey, Broccoli & Cheese	1	270	
Lightlife			
Tortilla Wrap, Mexican	1	340	
Tortilla Wrap, Ranchero	1	300	
Smart Ones—Smartwich			
Garden Veggies & Mozzarella	1	270	
Ham & Cheddar	1	270	
Pepperoni Pizza	1	290	
Three Cheese & Italian Meatball	1	290	
FRUIT SNACKS			
Betty Crocker Fruit by the Foot, all flavors	1 roll	80	
Betty Crocker Fruit Roll-Ups, all flavors	1 roll	50	
Betty Crocker Fruit Flavored Shapes	1 pkg	80	
GARLIC, raw	1 oz	42	
GELATIN			
Jell-O, all flavors, regular, prep	½ c	80	
Jell-O, all flavors, sugar free, prep	½ c	10	

Protein (g)	Total Fat (g)	Sat. Fat (g)	Trans Fat (g)	Chol. (mg)	Sodium (mg)	Calcium (%)	Iron (%)	Carbs (g)	Fiber (g)
11	7	4	0	20	810	20	15	43	3
12	7	3	0	30	620	12	10	44	3
13	20	7	0.5	20	880	25	15	40	3
10	14	5	0	30	770	20	15	42	3
12	7	3.5	0	25	590	20	10	41	3
7	4.5	1.5	0	45	310	8	10	19	2
12	7	3.5	0	45	630	25	15	42	3
12	7	3.5	0	25	530	15	15	40	3
16	7	1	0	0	630	na	na	54	7
15	6	1	0	0	370	na	na	48	7
14	6	2.5	0	20	570	20	15	40	3
14	6	3	0	30	650	8	15	40	1
16	7	2.5	1	25	700	15	6	41	2
15	7	2.5	0	20	650	15	10	43	3
0	1	0	0	0	50	0	0	17	0
0	1	0	0	0	55	0	0	12	0
0	0	0	0	0	50	0	0	21	0
2	0	0	0	0	5	5	3	9	1
2	0	0	0	0	80	0	0	19	0
1	0	0	0	0	60	0	0	0	0

Gelatin – Grapefruit Juice FOOD NAME	Portion Size	Calories	
Royal, all flavors, regular, prep	½ c	70	
Royal, all flavors, sugar free, prep	½ c	5	
GRAPES, green or red	1½ c	90	
GRAPE JUICE/DRINK			
Capri Sun, juice drink	8 oz	100	
Cascadian Farms, organic grape juice	8 oz	150	
Kool-Aid, sugar-sweetened	8 oz	60	
Kool-Aid, sugar-free	8 oz	5	
Welch's, light w/ calcium	8 oz	70	
Welch's, purple 100% juice	8 oz	170	
Welch's, white 100% juice	8 oz	160	
Welch's, white grape peach	8 oz	160	
GRAPEFRUIT			
Fresh, pink or red	½ fruit	52	
Fresh, white	½ fruit	39	
Del Monte, sections, red	½ c	90	
Del Monte, sun fresh red	½ c	80	
Del Monte, sun fresh white in real juice	½ c	45	
Fruit Naturals, red grapefruit	½ c	60	
GRAPEFRUIT JUICE			
Dole, ruby red 100% juice blend	11.5 oz	190	
Knudsen, organic	8 oz	100	
Knudsen, Rio Red	8 oz	140	
Minute Maid, 100% juice, frozen, w/ calcium	8 oz	100	
Tropicana, 100% juice, ruby red	8 oz	90	

Protein (g)	Total Fat (g)	Sat. Fat (g)	Trans Fat (g)	Chol. (mg)	Sodium (mg)	Calcium (%)	Iron (%)	Carbs (g)	Fiber (g)
1	0	0	0	0	115	0	0	17	0
1	0	0	0	0	70	0	0	0	0
1	1	0	0	0	0	2	2	24	1
0	0	0	0	0	15	0	0	25	0
0	0	0	0	0	5	0	0	38	0
0	0	0	0	0	0	0	0	16	0
0	0	0	0	0	0	0	0	10	0
0	0	0	0	0	80	10	0	18	0
0	0	0	0	0	20	0	0	42	0
0	0	0	0	0	20	0	0	39	0
0	0	0	0	0	15	0	0	89	0
1	0	0	0	0	0	3	1	13	2
1	0	0	0	0	0	1	0	10	1
1	0	0	0	0	0	2	15	21	1
1	0	0	0	0	10	2	0	19	2
1	0	0	0	0	15	2	10	9	2
0	0	0	0	0	15	2	0	16	<1
1	0	0	0	0	20	2	2	47	0
1	0	0	0	0	5	2	2	23	0
1	0	0	0	0	15	2	2	35	0
0	0	0	0	0	0	10	0	25	0
1	0	0	0	0	0	2	0	22	0

FOOD NAME	Portion Size	Calories	
Tropicana, sweet grapefruit	8 oz	130	
GRAVY			
Boston Market, Pan Style Beef	2 oz	40	
Boston Market, Pan Style Poultry	2 oz	40	
Campbell's			
Beef	¼ c	25	
Brown w/ Onions	¼ c	25	
Chicken Giblet	¼ c	30	
Chicken	¼ c	40	
Country Style Cream	¼ c	45	
Creamy Mushroom	¼ c	20	
Fat Free Beef	¼ c	15	
Fat Free Chicken	¼ c	15	
Golden Pork	¼ c	45	
Mushroom	¼ c	20	
Turkey	¼ c	25	
Franco-American, Beef	¼ c	25	
Franco-American, Turkey	¼ c	25	
Franco-American, f-f Slow Roast Beef	¼ c	20	
Franco-American, f-f Slow Roast Chicken	¼ c	20	
Heinz, Classic Chicken	¼ c	25	
GREEN BEANS			
Fresh, boiled, no salt	1 c	44	
Canned			
Del Monte, cut	½ c	20	

Protein (g)	Total Fat (g)	Sat. Fat (g)	Trans Fat (g)	Chol. (mg)	Sodium (mg)	Calcium (%)	Iron (%)	Carbs (g)	Fiber (g)
1	0	0	0	0	20	2	0	31	0
1	2.5	1	0	5	340	na	na	3	0
1	2	1	0	5	280	na	na	3	0
1	1	0.5	0	<5	270	0	0	3	0
0	1	0	0	0	330	0	0	4	0
1	1.5	0.5	0	10	300	0	0	3	0
0	3	1	0	5	260	0	0	3	0
1	3	1	0	5	190	0	0	3	0
0	0.5	0.5	0	<5	350	0	2	4	0
1	0	0	0	0	300	0	0	3	0
<1	0	0	0	<5	310	0	0	3	0
1	3	1.5	0	5	310	0	0	3	0
0	1	0	0	<5	280	0	0	3	0
1	1	0.5	0	0	270	0	0	3	0
1	1	0.5	0	5	270	0	0	3	0
1	1	0.5	0	0	270	0	0	3	0
1	0	0	0	<5	300	0	0	3	0
<1	0	0	0	<5	250	0	0	4	0
0	1	0	0	0	340	0	2	4	0
2	0	0	0	0	1	5	5	10	4
1	0	0	0	0	390	2	4	4	2

FOOD NAME	Portion Size	Calories	
Del Monte, cut Italian	½ c	30	
Del Monte, cut w/potatoes w/ ham style	½ c	30	
Del Monte, French style	½ c	20	
Del Monte, seasoned	½ c	20	
S&W, cut	½ c	20	
S&W, cut green & wax beans	½ c	20	
S&W, dilled green	½ c	20	
Frozen			
Cascadian Farms, cut, organic	¾ c	30	
Cascadian Farms, French w/almonds	⅔ c	70	
Green Giant, cut	½ c	20	
Green Giant, cut, low sodium	½ c	20	
Green Giant, French	½ c	20	
Green Giant, select whole	1 c	20	
Green Giant, green bean casserole	⅔ c	110	
Green Giant, green bean & garlic butter	½ c	50	
HADDOCK, baked	3 oz	95	
HALIBUT, Atlantic & Pacific, baked	3 oz	119	
Greenland, baked	3 oz	203	
HAM			
Cured, extra lean, roasted	3 oz	123	
Cured, regular	3 oz	151	
Fresh, leg, shank, lean & fat, roasted	3 oz	246	
Fresh, rump, lean & fat, roasted	3 oz	214	
Healthy Choice, smoked ham	2 oz	60	

Protein (g)	Total Fat (g)	Sat. Fat (g)	Trans Fat (g)	Chol. (mg)	Sodium (mg)	Calcium (%)	Iron (%)	Carbs (g)	Fiber (g)
1	0	0	0	0	390	2	4	6	3
1	0	0	0	0	330	2	2	6	<1
1	0	0	0	0	390	2	4	4	2
1	0	0	0	0	360	2	4	4	2
1	0	0	0	0	330	2	2	6	<1
1	0	0	0	0	390	2	4	4	2
0	0	0	0	0	125	0	0	5	1
2	0	0	0	0	0	4	4	6	2
3	3	0	0	0	180	6	6	8	2
<1	0	0	0	0	400	2	4	4	1
1	0	0	0	0	200	2	2	4	1
1	0	0	0	0	390	2	2	4	1
1	0	0	0	0	10	2	0	4	2
2	8	2.5	1	0	460	2	2	8	1
2	1	1	0	<5	390	4	4	8	2
21	1	0	0	63	74	4	6	0	0
23	2	0	0	35	59	5	5	0	0
16	15	3	0	50	88	0	4	0	0
18	5	2	0	45	1023	1	7	1	0
19	8	3	0	50	1275	1	6	0	0
22	17	6	0	78	50	1	5	0	0
25	12	4	0	82	53	1	5	0	0
9	1.5	0.5	0	30	430	0	2	2	0

FOOD NAME	Portion Size	Calories	
Healthy Choice, Virginia brand	2 oz	60	
Oscar Mayer, deli style, honey shaved	⅕ pkg	50	
Oscar Mayer, smoked shaved	⅕ pkg	45	
HAMBURGER MIX (mix only)			
Bacon Cheeseburger	½ c	190	
Beef Pasta	⅓ c	110	
Beef Taco	½ c	140	
Cheeseburger Macaroni	⅓ c	160	
Cheesy Enchilada	½ c	190	
Cheesy Italian Shells	½ c	150	
Chili Macaroni	⅓ c	130	
Double Cheese Pizza	½ c	150	
Italian Sausage	⅓ c	140	
Lasagna	⅔ c	120	
Philly Cheese Steak	½ c	150	
Ravioli & Cheese	½ c	150	
Rice Oriental	¼ c	140	
Salisbury	⅔ c	120	
Stroganoff	⅔ c	130	
Tomato Basil Penne	⅓ c	150	
Zesty Italian	⅓ c	140	
HEALTH BARS AND SHAKES			
Atkins Advantage			
Almond Brownie Bar	1	220	
Café Mocha Shake	1 can	160	

Protein (g)	Total Fat (g)	Sat. Fat (g)	Trans Fat (g)	Chol. (mg)	Sodium (mg)	Calcium (%)	Iron (%)	Carbs (g)	Fiber (g)
9	1.5	0.5	0	25	480	0	2	2	0
9	1	0.5	0	25	640	na	4	2	na
9	1	0	0	25	640	na	4	0	0
6	0	2	2	5	890	8	4	30	1
4	5	1	0	0	740	0	4	22	1
4	11	1.5	0	0	840	2	6	28	1
4	2.5	0.5	0.5	0	820	2	4	31	1
4	4	1	1	<5	670	4	6	36	<1
4	1	0.5	0	0	880	2	4	32	1
4	1	0	0	0	690	2	6	28	1
4	1.5	0.5	0	0	890	4	4	32	1
5	1.5	0.5	0	<5	840	4	4	26	1
4	0.5	0	0	0	840	na	4	26	1
4	5	2	1	0	820	2	4	22	1
5	1.5	0.5	0	0	880	2	6	31	1
3	0.5	0	0	0	930	4	6	31	na
4	1	0.5	0	0	740	2	4	24	1
4	2.5	1	1	<5	780	2	4	23	1
5	1	0	0	0	730	0	6	30	1
4	1	0	0	0	710	2	.6	30	1
20	9	4	0	5	105	25	10	22	7
16	9	1.5	0	5	110	40	20	4	2

Health Bars and Shakes FOOD NAME	Portion Size	Calories	
Caramel Chocolate Peanut Nougat Bar	1	150	
Caramel Fudge Brownie Bar	1	160	
Chocolate Coconut Bar	1	230	
Chocolate Delight Shake	1 can	170	
Chocolate Peanut Butter Bar	1	240	
Chocolate Royale Shake	1 can	170	
Creamy Vanilla Shake	1 can	170	
Golden Oats Granola Bar	1	210	
Strawberry Supreme Shake	1 can	170	
Vanilla Caramel Crème Shake	1 can	170	
Atkins Morning Start			
Apple Crisp Bar	1	180	
Chocolate Chip Bar	1	160	
Creamy Cinnamon Bun Bar	1	150	
Mixed Berry Bar	1	150	
Oatmeal Raisin Bar	1	140	
Strawberry Crisp Bar	1	160	
Balance Bars			
Almond Brownie, original	1	200	
Caramel & Chocolate, Carbwell	1	190	
Chewy Chocolate Chip, Gold	1	210	
Chocolate, original	1	200	
Chocolate Fudge, Carbwell	1	190	
Chocolate Peanut Butter, Carbwell	1	200	
Chocolate Peanut Butter, Gold	1	210	

Protein (g)	Total Fat (g)	Sat. Fat (g)	Trans Fat (g)	Chol. (mg)	Sodium (mg)	Calcium (%)	Iron (%)	Carbs (g)	Fiber (g)
11	7	3.5	0	5	130	30	10	17	9
12	8	5	0	<5	85	30	10	17	9
19	10	8	0	0	95	30	10	23	10
18	9	2	0	5	165	40	25	5	4
19	11	6	0	0	180	30	10	22	10
18	9	2	0	5	125	40	25	6	4
18	9	1.5	0	5	125	40	20	4	3
17	8	3.5	0	0	150	60	15	18	7
18	9	1.5	0	5	125	40	20	4	2
18	9	1.5	0	5	120	50	20	4	2
11	9	4.5	0	0	80	40	0	14	7
13	7	3.5	0	0	100	20	0	15	5
12	7	5	0	0	60	35	0	15	9
12	5	1	0	0	105	25	0	13	4
11	4	1	0	0	95	35	0	15	5
12	9	4.5	0	0	95	40	6	14	7
14	6	1.5	0	<5	115	10	25	23	2
14	7	4	0	<5	200	10	25	23	1
15	7	4	0	<5	140	10	25	22	<1
14	6	3.5	0	<5	180	10	25	22	<1
14	6	4	0	<5	190	10	25	23	2
14	8	4	0	<5	190	10	25	22	1
15	7	4	0	0	125	10	25	22	<1

Health Bars and Shakes FOOD NAME	Portion Size	Calories	
Cookie Dough, original	1	200	
Mocha Chip, original	1	200	
Rocky Road, Gold	1	210	
Yogurt Honey Peanut, original	1	200	
Clif Bar			
Banana Nut Bread	1	250	
Carrot Cake	1	240	
Chocolate Chip	1	250	
Crunch Peanut Butter	1	250	
Lemon Poppyseed	1	240	
Oatmeal Raisin Walnut	1	240	
Luna			
Caramel Nut Brownie	1	190	
Cherry Covered Chocolate	1	180	
Chocolate Peppermint Stick	1	180	
Cookies & Cream Delight	1	180	
Key Lime Pie	1	180	
Lemon Zest	1	180	
Peanut Butter Cookie	1	180	
S'mores	1	180	
Strawberries 'n Crème, Sunrise	1	180	
Vanilla Almond, Sunrise	1	180	
PowerBar, Harvest Whole Grain			
Dipped Double Chocolate Crisp	1	250	
Dipped Oatmeal Raisin	1	250	

Protein (g)	Total Fat (g)	Sat. Fat (g)	Trans Fat (g)	Chol. (mg)	Sodium (mg)	Calcium (%)	Iron (%)	Carbs (g)	Fiber (g)
15	6	3.5	0	<5	180	10	25	22	<1
14	6	3.5	0	0	125	10	25	23	<1
15	7	4	0	0	80	10	25	22	1
15	6	3	0	0	190	10	25	22	<1
10	6	1	0	0	130	25	25	43	5
10	4	1.5	0	0	150	25	25	46	5
10	5	2	0	0	150	25	25	45	5
12	6	1.5	0	0	250	25	25	40	5
10	3.5	1.5	0	0	110	25	25	46	5
10	5	1	0	0	130	25	25	43	5
9	6	3	0	0	125	35	35	27	4
9	5	3	0	0	150	35	35	28	3
9	5	3	0	0	130	35	35	27	1
10	4.5	3	0	0	130	35	35	27	2
10	4	3	0	0	150	35	35	26	3
10	4	3	0	0	150	35	35	26	3
10	6	3	0	0	120	35	35	25	3
10	5	3	0	0	125	35	35	26	3
8	4	2	0	0	95	35	20	29	5
8	4.5	2	0	0	95	35	20	29	5
10	5	2.5	0	0	140	40	25	42	5
10	5	2	0	0	140	40	25	42	5

FOOD NAME	Portion Size	Calories	
Heart Healthy Apple Cinnamon Crisp	1	240	
Heart Healthy Strawberry Crunch	1	240	
PowerBar Performance			
Apple Cinnamon	1	230	
Banana	1	230	
Chocolate Peanut Butter	1	240	
Oatmeal Raisin	1	230	
Vanilla Crisp	1	230	
Wild Berry	1	230	
PowerBar Pria 110 Plus			
Chocolate Peanut Crunch	1	110	
Double Chocolate Cookie	1	110	
French Vanilla Crisp	1	110	
Mint Chocolate Cookie	1	110	
PowerBar Protein Plus			
Chocolate Crisp	1	290	
Chocolate Peanut Butter	1	300	
Cookies & Cream	1	300	
Vanilla Yogurt	1	300	
PowerBar Triple Threat			
Caramel Peanut Fusion	1	230	
Caramel Peanut Crisp	1	220	
Chocolate Caramel	1	230	
Chocolate Peanut Butter Crisp	1	220	
Slim-Fast Optima Meal Bars			

Protein (g)	Total Fat (g)	Sat. Fat (g)	Trans Fat (g)	Chol. (mg)	Sodium (mg)	Calcium (%)	Iron (%)	Carbs (g)	Fiber (g)
10	4	0.5	0	0	140	40	25	42	5
10	4	0.5	0	0	140	40	25	42	5
9	2.5	0.5	0	0	100	30	35	45	3
9	2.5	0.5	0	0	100	30	35	45	3
10	3	1	0	0	95	30	35	45	3
10	2.5	0.5	0	0	110	30	35	45	3
9	2.5	0.5	0	0	90	30	35	45	3
9	2.5	0.5	0	0	95	30	35	45	3
5	3.5	2	0	0	85	30	20	16	1
5	3	2.5	0	0	100	30	20	16	1
5	3	2.5	0	0	80	30	20	17	1
5	3.5	2.5	0	0	90	30	20	15	1
23	6	3.5	0	0	190	45	45	37	2
23	6	3.5	0	0	210	40	45	39	1
23	6	3.5	0	0	170	40	45	38	1
23	6	3.5	0	0	150	45	45	38	1
10	8	4.5	0	0	190	15	15	30	4
11	5	2	0	0	210	15	15	32	4
10	8	4.5	0	0	150	15	15	30	4
11	5	2	0	0	180	15	30	32	4

Health Bars and Shakes – Herring, Atlantic, kippered FOOD NAME	Portion Size	Calories
Blueberry Crisp	1	180
Chocolate Chip Granola	1	220
Milk Chocolate Peanut	1	220
Oatmeal Raisin	1	220
Peanut Butter Chewy Granola	1	220
Rich Chocolate Brownie	1	220
Strawberry Cheesecake	1	220
Trail Mix Chewy Granola	1	210
Slim-Fast Optima Shakes		
Cappuccino Delight	1 can	180
Creamy Milk Chocolate	1 can	190
French Vanilla	1 can	180
Rich Chocolate Royale	1 can	190
Strawberry 'n Cream	1 can	180
Slim-Fast Optima Snack Bars		
Apple Cinnamon Muffin	1	140
Banana & Nut Muffin	1	150
Blueberry Muffin	1	140
Chocolate Mint Crisp	1	120
Chocolate Peanut Nougat	1	120
Crispy Peanut Caramel	1	120
Oatmeal Raisin Cookie	1	120
Peanut Butter Crunch	1	120
HERRING, Atlantic, kippered	1 oz	61
Atlantic, pickled	1 oz	74

Protein (g)	Total Fat (g)	Sat. Fat (g)	Trans Fat (g)	Chol. (mg)	Sodium (mg)	Calcium (%)	Iron (%)	Carbs (g)	Fiber (g)
8	4	2.5	0	0	150	25	15	28	3
8	6	3.5	0	<5	290	30	15	35	2
8	5	3	0	<5	160	30	15	34	3
8	5	3	0	<5	75	30	15	35	2
8	6	3	0	<5	360	30	15	35	2
8	5	3.5	0	<5	170	30	15	34	2
8	6	4	0	<5	130	30	15	34	2
8	5	1	0	<5	190	30	15	34	2
10	6	2	0	5	200	50	15	25	5
10	6	2.5	0	5	200	50	15	25	5
10	6	2.5	0	5	200	50	15	24	5
10	0	2.5	0	5	200	50	15	24	5
10	5	2	0	5	200	50	15	23	5
1	5	0.5	0	<5	180	25	15	21	1
2	8	0.5	0	<5	200	25	15	18	1
1	5	0.5	0	<5	170	25	15	22	1
2	4	3	0	5	100	25	15	19	<1
2	4	2.5	0	<5	70	25	15	20	1
1	4	3	0	<5	120	25	15	2	1
2	3.5	1.5	0	0	115	25	15	19	1
1	4	2	0	0	80	20	15	21	<1
7	3	1	0	23	259	2	2	0	0
4	5	1	0	4	246	2	2	3	0

Herring, Atlantic, Kippered – Ice Cream FOOD NAME	Portion Size	Calories	
Pacific, broiled	3 oz	212	
HONEY	1 Tbs	64	
HONEYDEW, raw, balls	1 c	64	
HORSERADISH, prep	1 Tbs	7	
Woeber's, sauce	1 tsp	20	
HUMMUS			
Athenos, Artichoke & Garlic	1 oz	45	
Athenos, Black Olive	1 oz	50	
Athenos, Cucumber Dill	1 oz	50	
Athenos, original	1 oz	50	
Athenos, Roasted Eggplant	1 oz	45	
Athenos, Roasted Garlic	1 oz	50	
Athenos, Roasted Red Pepper	1 oz	50	
Fantastic Foods	2 Tbs	60	
ICE CREAM			
Ben & Jerry's			
Black & Tan	½ c	230	
Butter Pecan	½ c	280	
Cherry Garcia	½ c	250	
Chocolate	½ c	260	
Chunky Monkey	½ c	300	
Coffee	½ c	240	
Fossil Fuel	½ c	280	
Half-baked	½ c	280	
Mint Chocolate Cookie	½ c	260	

Protein (g)	Total Fat (g)	Sat. Fat (g)	Trans Fat (g)	Chol. (mg)	Sodium (mg)	Calcium (%)	Iron (%)	Carbs (g)	Fiber (g)
18	15	4	0	84	81	9	7	0	0
0	0	0	0	0	1	0	0	17	0
1	3	0	0	0	32	1	2	16	1
<1	0	0	0	0	47	1	0	2	0
<1	1.5	0	0	<5	20	na	na	27	0
2	2.5	0	0	0	160	0	2	4	1
1	3	0	0	0	180	2	2	5	1
1	3	0	0	0	160	0	2	5	1
1	3	0	0	0	160	0	2	5	1
1	2	0	0	0	160	0	2	5	1
1	3	0	0	0	160	0	2	6	1
1	3	0	0	0	160	0	2	5	1
3	2	0	0	0	200	2	6	7	2
4	13	9	0	50	55	15	8	24	1
4	21	10	0	65	105	15	2	20	0
4	14	10	0	60	50	15	4	26	<1
4	16	11	0	50	50	15	6	25	2
5	18	10	0	55	45	15	4	30	1
4	15	10	0	75	60	15	2	21	0
4	18	12	0	55	60	15	4	31	1
5	14	9	0	50	90	10	10	34	<1
4	16	9	0	65	100	15	4	26	0

Ice Cream

FOOD NAME	Portion Size	Calories
New York Super Fudge Chunk	½ c	310
Neapolitan Dynamite	½ c	250
Turtle Soup	½ c	280
Vanilla Heath Bar Crunch	½ c	290
Vermonty Python	½ c	310
Breyers		
Butter Almond	½ c	160
Butter Pecan	½ c	160
Caramel Fudge	½ c	160
Caramel Praline	½ c	170
Cherry Vanilla	½ c	140
Chocolate	½ c	140
Chocolate Chip, natural	½ c	160
Chocolate Chip Cookie Dough	½ c	160
Cookies & Cream, natural	½ c	160
French Vanilla	½ c	140
Mint Chocolate Chip, natural	½ c	160
Peach	½ c	120
Rocky Road	½ c	160
Strawberry	½ c	120
Vanilla Fudge Brownie	½ c	150
Vanilla Fudge Twirl	½ c	130
Breyers, Double Churn		
Chocolate Caramel Brownie	½ c	160
Creamy Chocolate	½ c	140

Protein (g)	Total Fat (g)	Sat. Fat (g)	Trans Fat (g)	Chol. (mg)	Sodium (mg)	Calcium (%)	Iron (%)	Carbs (g)	Fiber (g)
5	20	11	0	40	55	15	6	29	2
4	13	9	0	45	70	10	6	29	1
4	15	10	0	30	100	15	4	60	0
4	18	11	1	65	120	15	2	29	0
4	19	11	0	60	90	15	4	30	1
3	10	4.5	0	20	100	10	0	15	0
3	10	4.5	0	20	110	10	0	14	0
3	7	4.5	0	20	75	8	0	20	0
3	7	4	0	20	110	10	0	22	0
3	6	4	0	20	40	10	0	17	0
3	8	4.5	0	20	30	8	2	17	0
3	8	6	0	20	40	10	2	17	0
3	8	5	0	20	50	10	0	20	0
3	8	5	0	20	85	10	0	19	0
3	8	5	0	50	45	10	0	15	0
3	8	5	0	20	40	10	2	17	0
2	5	3	0	15	30	8	0	17	0
3	8	4.5	0	20	60	8	2	20	1
2	5	3.5	0	15	30	8	0	15	0
3	7	4.5	0	15	50	10	4	20	0
3	6	4	0	20	50	10	2	17	0
3	7	4.5	0	15	80	8	4	22	0
3	7	4.5	0	20	35	8	2	17	0

Ice Cream FOOD NAME	Portion Size	Calories	
Strawberries & Cream	½ c	130	
Vanilla, Chocolate, Strawberry	½ c	140	
98% f-f Vanilla	½ c	90	
Dreyer's—Grand			
Almond Praline	½ c	150	
Butter Pecan	½ c	170	
Chocolate	½ c	150	
Cookie Dough	½ c	180	
Fudge Tracks	½ c	180	
Mocha Almond Fudge	½ c	160	
Peanut Butter Cup	½ c	180	
Rocky Road	½ c	170	
Spumoni	½ c	150	
Toffee Bar Crunch	½ c	170	
Turtle Sundae	½ c	160	
Dreyer's—Slow Churned Light			
Butter Pecan	½ c	120	
Chocolate Chip	½ c	120	
Cookies & Cream	½ c	120	
Mint Chocolate Chip	½ c	120	
Neapolitan	½ c	100	
Peanut Butter Cup	½ c	130	
Rocky Road	½ c	120	
Strawberry	½ c	110	
Vanilla Bean	½ c	100	

Protein (g)	Total Fat (g)	Sat. Fat (g)	Trans Fat (g)	Chol. (mg)	Sodium (mg)	Calcium (%)	Iron (%)	Carbs (g)	Fiber (g)
2	6	3.5	0	15	35	8	0	16	0
3	7	4.5	0	20	40	8	0	17	0
3	1.5	1	0	5	55	10	0	19	0
2	7	4	0	25	85	4	na	20	na
3	10	4.5	0	25	95	6	na	16	na
3	8	4.5	0	25	35	6	na	17	na
3	9	6	0	25	55	6	na	21	na
3	11	6	0	25	60	6	na	18	na
3	9	4.5	0	25	45	6	na	17	na
3	10	4	0	20	75	6	na	19	na
3	10	5	0	30	35	6	na	19	na
3	8	4.5	0	25	40	6	na	16	na
2	9	5	0	25	65	6	na	19	na
3	9	4.5	0	25	50	6	na	18	na
3	5	2	0	20	80	6	na	16	na
3	4.5	3	0	20	50	6	na	17	na
3	4	2	0	20	60	6	na	18	na
3	4.5	3	0	20	50	6	na	17	na
3	3	2	0	20	40	6	na	15	na
3	6	3	0	20	65	6	na	17	na
3	4	2	0	20	40	6	na	17	na
3	3	1.5	0	15	40	6	na	18	na
3	3.5	2	0	20	45	6	na	15	na

Ice Cream – Ice Cream Novelties FOOD NAME	Portion Size	Calories	
Vanilla Chocolate	½ c	100	
Häagen-Dazs—Regular			
Bailey's Irish Cream	½ c	270	
Banana Split	½ c	280	
Black Walnut	½ c	300	
Butter Pecan	½ c	310	
Cherry Vanilla	½ c	240	
Chocolate	½ c	270	
Chocolate Peanut Butter	½ c	360	
English Toffee	½ c	350	
Rocky Road	½ c	300	
Strawberry Cheesecake	½ c	260	
Vanilla Fudge Brownie	½ c	300	
Häagen-Dazs—Light			
Blueberry Cheesecake	½ c	230	
Cherry Fudge Truffle	½ c	230	
Cookies & Cream	½ c	210	
Mint Chip	½ c	230	
Vanilla Caramel Brownie	½ c	240	
ICE CREAM NOVELTIES			
Dreyer's			
Dibs, Caramel w/ Chocolate Coating	26 pcs	440	
Dibs, Cookies & Cream w/ Chocolate Coating	26 pcs	410	
Dibs, Peanut Butter w/ Chocolate Coating	26 pcs	510	

Protein (g)	Total Fat (g)	Sat. Fat (g)	Trans Fat (g)	Chol. (mg)	Sodium (mg)	Calcium (%)	Iron (%)	Carbs (g)	Fiber (g)
3	3.5	2	0	20	45	6	na	15	na
5	17	10	0.5	115	70	15	0	23	0
4	16	9	0	90	70	10	2	31	0
5	22	11	0.5	105	85	10	2	21	0
5	23	11	0	110	110	15	2	21	1
4	15	9	0.5	100	60	10	0	23	0
5	18	11	0.5	115	60	15	6	22	1
8	24	11	0	100	100	10	10	27	2
4	22	13	0.5	110	150	10	0	33	0
5	18	9	0	90	75	10	8	29	1
4	15	8	0.5	95	80	8	0	27	0
5	19	11	0	105	100	8	4	25	0
5	7	4.5	0	60	115	10	2	36	0
5	7	4	0	50	40	10	2	37	0
6	6	3.5	0	45	30	10	2	33	0
6	8	5	0	55	65	15	2	34	0
6	7	4	0	50	75	15	0	37	0
3	32	22	0	20	80	10	na	35	na
4	29	20	0	20	95	10	na	33	na
7	39	23	0	20	170	8	na	32	na

Ice Cream Novelties FOOD NAME	Portion Size	Calories	
Dibs, Vanilla w/ Chocolate Coating	26 pcs	420	
Dibs, Vanilla w/ Nestlé Crunch	26 pcs	380	
Fruit Bars: Creamy Coconut	1	130	
Fruit Bars: Grape	1	80	
Fruit Bars: Orange & Cream	1	80	
Fruit Bars: Strawberry	1	80	
Good Humor			
Chocolate Éclair Bar	1	160	
Cone, Oreo Cookies & Cream	1	220	
Cone, Premium Sundae	1	260	
Cone, Vanilla King	1	250	
Cyclone Caramel Tracks	1	500	
Cyclone Chocolate Chip Cookie Dough	1	570	
Cyclone Cookies & Cream	1	540	
Strawberry Shortcake Bar	1	170	
Toasted Almond Bar	1	180	
Häagen-Dazs			
Brownie Bar	1	360	
Chocolate & Dark Chocolate Bar	1	300	
Coffee & Almond Crunch	1	310	
Mint & Dark Chocolate	1	290	
Vanilla & Milk Chocolate	1	290	
Klondike			
Bar, Chocolate	1	250	
Bar, Heath	1	270	

Protein (g)	Total Fat (g)	Sat. Fat (g)	Trans Fat (g)	Chol. (mg)	Sodium (mg)	Calcium (%)	Iron (%)	Carbs (g)	Fiber (g)
3	32	19	0	25	65	8	na	29	na
3	28	20	0	25	90	8	na	29	na
3	3	2.5	0	0	40	8	na	22	na
0	0	0	0	0	0	na	na	20	na
1	1.5	0.5	0	5	30	4	na	16	na
0	0	0	0	0	0	na	na	21	na
2	8	3.5	0	5	55	4	4	21	1
3	10	6	0	15	120	6	6	32	1
4	15	9	0	15	80	6	2	29	1
4	13	8	0	15	100	8	4	30	1
6	23	16	0.5	50	300	25	2	67	1
6	20	18	0.5	50	220	20	8	74	2
7	28	13	2	45	210	20	4	68	2
1	9	2.5	2	5	60	2	0	21	0
2	10	2.5	2	10	30	4	0	22	1
5	24	13	0	80	95	10	6	30	1
4	21	13	0	70	40	8	6	24	<1
4	22	12	0	75	65	10	4	23	<1
4	20	12	0	65	30	8	6	23	1
4	21	14	0	75	55	10	4	22	0
3	17	13	0	20	45	8	4	21	0
2	19	13	0.5	20	80	8	0	24	0

FOOD NAME	Portion Size	Calories	
Ice Cream Novelties – Ice Cream Substitutes (Non-Dairy)			
Bar, Krunch	1	250	
Bar, Oreo	1	260	
Bar, Reese's	1	270	
Bar, Vanilla	1	250	
Cone, Vanilla	1	280	
Cone, Vanilla Fudge	1	300	
Sandwich, Ice Cream Cookie	1	260	
Sandwich, Vanilla	1	190	
Slim-A-Bear, Cookies & Cream	1	110	
Slim-A-Bear, Krunch	1	170	
Slim-A-Bear, Vanilla	1	170	
Slim-A-Bear, Vanilla Sandwich	1	130	
Popsicle			
Creamsicle	1.65 oz	70	
Creamsicle, sugar free	1	40	
Fudgsicle	1.65 oz	60	
Tropicals, sugar free	1	15	
ICE CREAM SUBSTITUTES (Non-Dairy)			
Soy Delicious—Organic			
Butter Pecan	½ c	260	
Chocolate Velvet	½ c	130	
Creamy Vanilla	½ c	130	
Mocha Fudge	½ c	130	
Peanut Butter	½ c	150	
Soy Delicious—Novelties			

Protein (g)	Total Fat (g)	Sat. Fat (g)	Trans Fat (g)	Chol. (mg)	Sodium (mg)	Calcium (%)	Iron (%)	Carbs (g)	Fiber (g)
3	17	13	0	20	70	8	0	22	0
3	17	11	1	15	120	6	6	26	0
3	18	11	0	15	90	8	2	24	1
3	17	13	0	20	55	10	0	22	0
5	16	9	0	15	85	8	2	30	1
5	16	10	0	15	110	8	4	35	1
3	11	5	0	15	220	4	8	38	1
3	7	3.5	0.5	15	105	6	0	29	0
5	16	10	0	15	110	8	2	25	3
4	10	8	0	5	85	15	2	22	4
4	9	8	0	5	65	15	0	21	4
3	1.5	0	0	5	95	10	2	29	3
1	1.5	1	0	5	20	2	0	12	0
1	2	1.5	0	0	5	2	0	10	0
1	1.5	1.5	0	0	45	4	2	12	0
0	0	0	0	0	0	na	na	4	0
2	7	1	0	0	90	0	2	22	3
2	3.5	0.5	0	0	50	0	4	23	1
1	3	0	0	0	55	0	2	24	3
2	3	0	0	0	85	0	8	26	3
3	6	1	0	0	80	0	2	23	3

FOOD NAME	Portion Size	Calories	
Ice Cream Substitutes (Non-Dairy)			
Li'l Buddies, Chocolate	1	150	
Li'l Buddies, Vanilla	1	180	
So Delicious Dairy-Free Bars, Orange	1	80	
So Delicious Dairy-Free Bars, Fudge	1	80	
Sweet Nothings, Fudge Bar	1	100	
Sweet Nothings, Mango Raspberry	1	100	
Tofutti			
Better Pecan	½ c	210	
Chocolate Fudge, low-fat	½ c	145	
Chocolate Cookie Crunch	½ c	190	
Chocolate Supreme	½ c	180	
Coffee Marshmallow Swirl, low-fat	½ c	120	
Vanilla	½ c	190	
Vanilla Fudge	½ c	190	
Tofutti Cheesecake Supreme, Chocolate, Blueberry, or Strawberry	½ c	200	
Tofutti—Cuties			
Chocolate	1	130	
Coffee Break	1	130	
Cookies & Cream	1	120	
Peanut Butter	1	165	
Totally Vanilla	1	120	
Vanilla	1	120	
Tofutti Super Soy, Bella Vanilla	½ c	160	
Tofutti Super Soy, New York Chocolate	½ c	170	

Protein (g)	Total Fat (g)	Sat. Fat (g)	Trans Fat (g)	Chol. (mg)	Sodium (mg)	Calcium (%)	Iron (%)	Carbs (g)	Fiber (g)
3	4.5	2	0	0	25	2	6	28	3
3	4.5	2	0	0	30	2	6	28	3
1	1.5	0	0	0	30	10	0	18	2
1	2	0	0	0	30	10	2	18	2
1	0	0	0	0	5	0	0	23	0
1	0	0	0	0	0	0	0	23	0
1	13	2	0	0	200	na	na	22	0
2	4	1	0	0	98	na	na	25	0
3	11	2	0	0	100	na	na	26	0
3	11	2	0	0	180	na	na	18	0
1	30	0	0		77	na	na	24	0
2	11	2	0	0	210	na	na	20	0
2	9	2	0	0	130	na	na	25	0
2	12	2	0	0	200	na	na	20	0
2	5	1	0	0	110	na	na	16	0
2	5	1	0	0	110	na	na	16	0
2	6	1	0	0	135	na	na	17	0
3	8	2	0	0	135	na	na	20	0
2	5	1	0	0	110	na	na	16	0
2	5	1	0	0	121	na	na	17	0
4	8	0	0	0	190	na	na	20	0
4	9	0	0	0	180	na	na	22	0

FOOD NAME	Portion Size	Calories	
JAM, JELLY, PRESERVES			
Cascadian Farm Fruit Spreads, organic			
Apricot, Concord Grape, or Strawberry	1 Tbs	40	
Blackberry, Blueberry, or Raspberry	1 Tbs	45	
Smucker's Jam: Concord Grape	1 Tbs	50	
Smucker's Jam, Red Plum	1 Tbs	50	
Smucker's Jelly, all flavors	1 Tbs	50	
Smucker's Simply Fruit, all	1 Tbs	40	
Welch's Grape Jelly	1 Tbs	50	
Welch's Jam, Marmalade	1 Tbs	50	
KALE, fresh, cooked, no salt, chopped	1 c	36	
KETCHUP			
Del Monte	1 Tbs	15	
Hunt's	1 Tbs	15	
KIELBASA			
Hillshire, Polska	2 oz	180	
Hillshire, Turkey	2 oz	90	
Jennie-O, Turkey	2 oz	70	
KNOCKWURST, Hebrew National Beef	1 link	260	
KUMQUAT, raw	1	13	
LAMB			
Australian, sirloin chop, lean, broiled	3 oz	160	
Australian, leg, whole, lean, roasted	3 oz	162	
Australian shoulder blade, lean & fat,			
broiled	3 oz	247	

Protein (g)	Total Fat (g)	Sat. Fat (g)	Trans Fat (g)	Chol. (mg)	Sodium (mg)	Calcium (%)	Iron (%)	Carbs (g)	Fiber (g)
0	0	0	0	0	0	0	0	10	0
0	0	0	0	0	0	0	0	11	0
0	0	0	0	0	0	0	0	13	0
0	0	0	0	0	5	0	0	13	0
0	0	0	0	0	0	0	0	13	0
0	0	0	0	0	0	0	0	10	0
0	0	0	0	0	1	0	0	13	0
0	0	0	0	0	10	0	0	13	0
2	1	0	0	0	30	9	7	30	3
0	0	0	0	0	190	0	0	4	0
0	0	0	0	0	100	0	0	4	0
6	15	6	0	35	620	0	2	2	0
8	5	2	0	35	560	0	2	2	0
9	3	1	0	35	550	2	4	1	0
10	24	11	0	55	670	0	6	1	0
0	0	0	0	0	2	1	1	3	1
23	7	3	0	72	56	1	12	0	0
23	7	3	0	76	61	1	10	0	0
18	19	9	0	71	75	2	7	0	0

Lamb – Lettuce		
FOOD NAME	Portion Size	Calories
Domestic, leg, sirloin half, lean & fat	3 oz	241
Domestic, loin, lean, roasted	3 oz	172
Domestic, rib, lean & fat, roasted	3 oz	290
New Zealand, frozen, loin, lean & fat, broiled	3 oz	252
New Zealand, frozen, rib, lean, roasted	3 oz	167
New Zealand, frozen, shoulder, lean & fat, braised	3 oz	291
LEMON, raw, peeled	1 c	61
LEMONADE		
Country Time, Regular & Pink	8 oz	60
Country Time, Strawberry	8 oz	80
Crystal Light, sugar free	8 oz	5
Kool-Aid, sugar sweetened	8 oz	70
Kool-Aid, unsweetened	8 oz	0
Minute Maid (carton)	8 oz	110
Minute Maid (frozen) Country Style	8 oz	110
Minute Maid (carton), Raspberry Lemonade	8 oz	120
Newman's Own Old Fashioned Roadside	8 oz	110
LENTILS, cooked, no salt	1 c	230
LETTUCE		
Butterhead (Boston, Bibb), shredded	1 c	7
Green Leaf, shredded	1 c	5
Iceberg, shredded	1 c	8
Red Leaf, shredded	1 c	4
Romaine, shredded	1 c	8

Protein (g)	Total Fat (g)	Sat. Fat (g)	Trans Fat (g)	Chol. (mg)	Sodium (mg)	Calcium (%)	Iron (%)	Carbs (g)	Fiber (g)
21	17	7	0	82	58	1	9	0	0
23	8	3	0	74	56	1	12	0	0
19	23	10	0	82	63	2	8	0	0
21	18	9	0	96	43	2	10	0	0
21	9	4	0	80	41	1	9	0	0
25	20	10	0	105	44	2	10	0	0
2	1	0	0	0	4	6	7	20	6
0	0	0	0	0	25	0	0	16	0
0	0	0	0	0	0	0	0	20	0
0	0	0	0	0	10	0	0	0	0
0	0	0	0	0	0	0	0	17	0
0	0	0	0	0	10	0	0	0	0
0	0	0	0	0	0	0	0	29	0
0	0	0	0	0	15	0	0	31	0
0	0	0	0	0	15	0	0	32	0
0	0	0	0	0	40	0	0	27	0
8	1	0	0	0	4	4	37	40	16
1	0	0	0	0	3	2	4	1	0
0	0	0	0	0	10	1	2	1	0
0	0	0	0	0	6	1	1	2	1
0	0	0	0	0	0	1	2	7	0
1	0	0	0	0	4	2	3	2	1

Lima Beans, fresh, boiled, no salt – Lunchables FOOD NAME	Portion Size	Calories	
LIMA BEANS, fresh, boiled, no salt	1 c	209	
Birds Eye, Baby Limas (frozen)	½ c	110	
Birds Eye, Fordhook (frozen)	½ c	100	
Del Monte, canned	½ c	80	
Green Giant, Baby Limas (frozen)	½ c	80	
Green Giant, Baby Limas & Butter	⅔ c	110	
LIME, fresh	1	20	
LIVER (see Beef, Chicken, Duck, Goose)			
LIVERWURST, Oscar Mayer Braunschweiger	2 oz	190	
LOBSTER			
Northern, cooked	3 oz	83	
Spiny, cooked	3 oz	122	
LUNCHABLES			
Bologna & American Cracker Stackers	1 pkg	390	
Chicken Dunks	1 pkg	300	
Chicken Shakeups, BBQ	1 pkg	210	
Chicken Strips, Maxed Out	1 pkg	480	
Ham & American Cracker Stackers	1 pkg	420	
Ham & cheese Cracker Stackers	1 pkg	400	
Ham & Swiss	1 pkg	340	
Ham & Swiss, low fat, Cracker Stackers	1 pkg	340	
Mini Burgers, grilled	1 pkg	410	
Mini Hot Dogs	1 pkg	400	
Nachos	1 pkg	380	
Pepperoni Pizza	1 pkg	310	

Protein (g)	Total Fat (g)	Sat. Fat (g)	Trans Fat (g)	Chol. (mg)	Sodium (mg)	Calcium (%)	Iron (%)	Carbs (g)	Fiber (g)
12	1	0	0	0	29	5	23	29	9
6	0	0	0	0	240	4	8	20	5
6	0	0	0	0	5	0	10	18	4
4	0	0	0	0	390	2	8	15	4
4	0	0	0	0	170	2	6	15	3
5	1.5	1	0	<5	390	0	6	20	4
0	0	0	0	0	1	2	2	7	2
8	17	6	0	90	630	na	na	1	0
17	1	0	0	61	323	5	2	1	0
22	2	0	0	77	193	5	7	3	0
14	22	9	1	60	890	25	10	34	1
13	5	1	0	25	560	2	8	51	0
13	6	2	0	25	490	10	6	28	1
14	13	3.5	1	30	890	6	15	73	1
14	17	9	0.5	45	780	25	8	54	1
16	20	9	1	50	930	20	10	40	1
20	17	9	1	65	1100	35	8	24	1
16	9	4	0	35	970	35	8	50	0
14	4	9	0.5	35	1000	20	15	56	1
10	12	4	0	30	690	15	15	63	1
7	21	6	0	10	830	0	0	41	1
16	11	4	0	30	570	30	4	37	3

Lunchables – Macaroni & Cheese (boxed, mix) FOOD NAME	Portion Size	Calories	
Pizza Cracker Stackers	1 pkg	420	
Pizza Extra Cheesy	1 pkg	310	
Pizza Stix, Maxed Out	1 pkg	680	
Pizza & Treatza	1 pkg	460	
Sub Sandwich, Ham, Turkey, Cheddar	1 pkg	460	
Taco Beef	1 pkg	460	
Turkey & American Cracker Stackers	1 pkg	390	
Turkey & Cheddar	1 pkg	340	
Turkey & Cheddar, Cracker Stackers	1 pkg	380	
Turkey, Ham, Swiss, Cheddar	1 pkg	360	
LUNCHEON LOAF			
Oscar Mayer, Ham & Cheese Loaf	1 oz	60	
Oscar Mayer, Luncheon Loaf Spiced	1 oz	60	
Oscar Mayer, Olive Loaf	1 oz	70	
Oscar Mayer, Pickle & Pimento Loaf	1 oz	80	
MACADAMIA NUTS, dry roasted, no salt	1 oz	203	
MACARONI (see "Pasta")			
MACARONI & CHEESE (boxed, mix) (also see "Pasta" and "Frozen Dinners")			
Kraft Deluxe w/ Original Cheddar Cheese	3.5 oz	320	
Kraft Deluxe Sharp Cheddar	3.5 oz	320	
Kraft Dinner Deluxe ½ the Fat	2 oz	290	
Kraft Dinner Deluxe Four Cheese Sauce	3.5 oz	320	
Kraft Premium Cheesy Alfredo	2 oz	260	
Kraft Premium Thick n' Creamy	2 oz	250	

Protein (g)	Total Fat (g)	Sat. Fat (g)	Trans Fat (g)	Chol. (mg)	Sodium (mg)	Calcium (%)	Iron (%)	Carbs (g)	Fiber (g)
6	18	8	0.5	50	970	25	8	50	1
17	10	4.5	0	25	600	45	2	37	3
20	10	4.5	0	15	1440	40	20	130	3
14	10	4.5	0	15	510	35	6	79	4
19	20	7	0.5	45	1450	35	20	52	2
20	12	5	0	40	1190	35	15	69	2
13	19	9	1	45	900	20	15	39	1
18	20	9	1	65	1140	30	8	23	1
12	13	6	0.5	45	780	20	6	57	1
20	19	9	1	70	1750	30	10	26	1
4	4.5	2.5	0	20	350	0	0	1	0
4	4.5	1.5	0	15	360	0	2	3	0
3	5	1.5	0	15	320	2	2	2	0
3	6	2	0	20	360	4	4	2	0
2	21	3	0	0	1	2	4	4	2
13	10	3.5	0	15	910	15	15	44	2
12	10	3.5	0	15	880	15	10	45	1
13	4.5	2.5	0	15	870	20	10	49	1
12	10	3.5	0	15	920	15	10	44	1
9	2.5	1	0	5	650	8	10	49	2
9	2	1	0	5	580	10	10	50	2

Macaroni & Cheese – Margarine & Spreads (boxed, mix) FOOD NAME	Portion Size	Calories	
Kraft Premium Three Cheese	2 oz	260	
Kraft Rotini & White Cheddar w/ Broccoli	4.4 oz	390	
Kraft The Cheesiest	2 oz	260	
MACKEREL			
Atlantic, broiled	3 oz	223	
King, broiled	3 oz	114	
Pacific, broiled	3 oz	171	
Spanish, broiled	3 oz	134	
w/ Tomato Sauce (Chicken of the Sea)	¼ c	70	
MANGO, fresh, sliced	1 c	107	
MARGARINE & SPREADS			
Benecol, regular	1 Tbs	70	
Benecol, light	1 Tbs	50	
Blue Bonnet, regular stick	1 Tbs	80	
Blue Bonnet, light stick	1 Tbs	50	
Blue Bonnet, homestyle soft	1 Tbs	60	
Blue Bonnet, homestyle, light, soft	1 Tbs	40	
Country Crock, regular, tub & sticks	1 Tbs	60	
Country Crock, churn style	1 Tbs	80	
Country Crock, light	1 Tbs	50	
Country Crock plus calcium	1 Tbs	50	
Fleischmann's, light, soft	1 Tbs	40	
Fleischmann's, w/ olive oil, soft tub	1 Tbs	70	
Fleischmann's, original, soft	1 Tbs	70	
I Can't Believe It's Not Butter, f-f	1 Tbs	5	

Protein (g)	Total Fat (g)	Sat. Fat (g)	Trans Fat (g)	Chol. (mg)	Sodium (mg)	Calcium (%)	Iron (%)	Carbs (g)	Fiber (g)
9	2.5	1	0	5	610	10	10	49	2
16	15	5	0	25	1470	25	15	48	2
9	2.5	1.5	0	10	600	20	10	48	1
20	15	4	0	64	71	1	7	0	0
22	2	0	0	58	173	3	11	0	0
22	9	2	0	51	93	2	7	0	0
20	5	2	0	62	56	1	3	0	0
10	3	1	0	45	250	15	6	2	0
1	0	0	0	0	3	2	1	28	3
0	8	1	0	0	110	na	na	0	0
0	5	0.5	0	0	110	na	na	0	0
0	9	2	1.5	0	110	na	na	0	0
0	5	1	0.5	0	80	na	na	0	0
0	7	1	0	0	125	na	na	0	0
0	4.5	1	0	0	90	na	na	0	0
0	7	1.5	1	0	110	na	na	0	0
0	8	1.5	1.5	0	95	na	na	0	0
0	5	1.5	0	0	85	na	na	0	0
0	5	1.5	0	0	85	10	na	0	0
0	4.5	0	0	0	90	na	na	0	0
0	8	1.5	0	0	95	na	na	0	0
0	8	1.5	0	0	75	na	na	0	0
0	0	0	0	0	90	na	na	0	0

Margarine & Spreads – Mayonnaise & Salad Dressing FOOD NAME	Portion Size	Calories	
I Can't Believe It's Not Butter, light, soft	1 Tbs	50	
I Can't Believe It's Not Butter, orig., soft	1 Tbs	80	
I Can't Believe It's Not Butter, spray	5 sprays	0	
Parkay, light, tub	1 Tbs	50	
Parkay, original stick	1 Tbs	90	
Parkay original soft, tub	1 Tbs	60	
Promise Buttery Spread, soft, light	1 Tbs	45	
Promise Buttery Spread, soft	1 Tbs	80	
Smart Balance, 67% light spread	1 Tbs	80	
Smart Balance, 37% light spread	1 Tbs	45	
Smart Balance Omega Plus	1 Tbs	80	
MARSHMALLOWS			
Jet-puffed Crème	½ oz	45	
Jet-puffed, Funmallows	1 oz	100	
Jet-pufffed, Toasted Coconut	1 oz	100	
MAYONNAISE & SALAD DRESSING			
Hellman's Canola	1 Tbs	90	
Hellman's Light	1 Tbs	45	
Hellman's Real Mayonnaise	1 Tbs	90	
Kraft f-f	1 Tbs	10	
Kraft, light	1 Tbs	40	
Kraft, Real Mayonnaise	1 Tbs	100	
Miracle Whip, f-f	1 Tbs	25	
Miracle Whip, light	1 Tbs	25	
Miracle Whip Dressing	1 Tbs	40	

Protein (g)	Total Fat (g)	Sat. Fat (g)	Trans Fat (g)	Chol. (mg)	Sodium (mg)	Calcium (%)	Iron (%)	Carbs (g)	Fiber (g)
0	5	1	0	0	85	na	na	0	0
0	8	2	0	0	90	na	na	0	0
0	0	0	0	0	15	0	0	0	0
0	5	1	0	0	130	na	na	0	0
0	10	2	2	0	105	na	na	0	0
0	7	1.5	0	0	100	na	na	0	0
0	5	1	0	0	85	na	na	0	0
0	8	1.5	0	0	85	na	na	0	0
0	9	2.5	0	0	90	na	na	0	0
0	5	1.5	0	0	90	na	na	0	0
0	9	2.5	0	0	90	na	na	0	0
0	0	0	0	na	10	na	na	11	0
1	0	0	0	na	15	na	na	24	0
1	2.5	2	0	na	20	na	na	21	0
0	10	1	0	5	90	na	na	0	0
0	4.5	0.5	0	<5	120	na	na	0	0
0	10	1.5	0	5	90	na	na	0	0
0	0	0	0	0	120	0	0	2	0
0	3.5	0.5	0	5	90	0	0	2	0
0	11	2	0	5	75	na	na	0	0
0	1.5	0	0	5	140	0	0	3	0
0	1.5	0	0	5	140	0	0	3	0
0	3.5	0.5	0	5	125	0	0	2	0

FOOD NAME	Portion Size	Calories	
Mayonnaise & Salad Dressing – Mixed Fruit			
Smart Balance Omega Plus Light Mayo	1 Tbs	50	
MILK			
1%, protein fortified	1 c	118	
2%, protein fortified	1 c	138	
Buttermilk, low-fat	1 c	98	
Chocolate, 2% (Organic Valley)	1 c	170	
Evaporated nonfat	½ c	100	
Evaporated, whole	½ c	169	
Hershey's 1% Chocolate Milk	1 c	120	
Lactose-free low-fat (Organic Valley)	1 c	110	
Lactaid, f-f	1 c	80	
Lactaid, 2%	1 c	130	
Skim, calcium fortified	1 c	86	
Whole	1 c	146	
MIXED FRUIT			
Del Monte			
Cherry Mixed	½ c	90	
Chunky Mixed	½ c	100	
Fruit Cocktail	½ c	100	
Fruit Naturals, Tropical Medley	½ c	70	
Lite Chunky Mixed	½ c	60	
Lite Fruit Cocktail	½ c	60	
Orchard Select, Premium Mixed	½ c	80	
Tropical Fruit Salad	½ c	60	
Dole			

Protein (g)	Total Fat (g)	Sat. Fat (g)	Trans Fat (g)	Chol. (mg)	Sodium (mg)	Calcium (%)	Iron (%)	Carbs (g)	Fiber (g)
0	5	0	0	5	125	na	na	0	0
10	3	2	0	10	143	35	1	14	0
10	5	3	0	20	145	35	1	14	0
8	2	1	0	10	257	28	1	12	0
8	5	3	0	20	250	30	4	23	<1
10	0	0	0	5	147	37	2	15	0
9	10	6	0	37	134	33	1	13	0
11	2.5	2	0	5	170	60	2	15	1
8	2.5	1.5	0	10	125	30	0	14	0
8	0	0	0	5	125	30	0	13	0
8	5	3	0	20	125	30	0	12	0
8	0	0	0	5	128	50	1	12	0
8	8	5	0	24	98	na	na	28	0
<1	0	0	0	0	10	0	0	22	<1
0	0	0	0	0	10	0	2	24	1
0	0	0	0	0	10	0	2	24	1
<1	0	0	0	0	5	0	0	18	<1
0	0	0	0	0	10	0	2	15	1
0	0	0	0	0	10	0	2	15	1
<1	0	0	0	0	10	0	0	20	<1
0	0	0	0	0	15	4	4	16	1

Mixed Fruit – Muffins (box/pouch mixes) FOOD NAME	Portion Size	Calories	
Mixed, frozen	¾ c	60	
Tropical Mixed	½ c	90	
S&W			
Chunky Mixed, natural style	½ c	80	
Cocktail, lite syrup	½ c	70	
Cocktail, natural style	½ c	80	
MOLASSES, Blackstrap	1 Tbs	47	
Regular	1 Tbs	58	
MOUSSE			
Dr. Oetker, Dark Chocolate Truffle, mix	2 Tbs	100	
Dr. Oetker, French Vanilla, mix	2 Tbs	90	
Dr. Oetker, Strawberry, mix	2 Tbs	80	
Nestlé Chocolate Raspberry Truffle	¼ pkg	90	
Nestlé Dark Chocolate	¼ pkg	80	
Nestlé Milk Chocolate	¼ pkg	80	
MUFFINS (box/pouch mixes)			
Betty Crocker			
Apple Streusel, mix	¼ c	160	
Authentic Cornbread & Muffin	3 Tbs	110	
Banana Nut, mix	3 Tbs	150	
Chocolate Chip, pouch	⅕ pkg	160	
Cinnamon Streusel	1/12 pkg	150	
Double Chocolate	1/12 pkg	190	
Lemon Poppy Seed	1/12 pkg	140	
Lemon Poppy Seed, pouch	⅙ pkg	130	

Protein (g)	Total Fat (g)	Sat. Fat (g)	Trans Fat (g)	Chol. (mg)	Sodium (mg)	Calcium (%)	Iron (%)	Carbs (g)	Fiber (g)
0	0	0	0	0	0	0	2	16	2
0	0	0	0	0	10	0	2	21	0
<1	0	0	0	0	20	0	0	19	3
0	0	0	0	0	15	0	0	18	1
0	0	0	0	0	20	0	2	20	2
0	0	0	0	0	11	17	19	12	0
0	0	0	0	0	7	4	5	15	0
2	3.5	3	0	0	85	0	4	15	1
0	3	2.5	0	0	130	na	na	15	0
0	3	2.5	0	0	140	na	na	13	0
0	2.5	1.5	0	0	30	2	0	14	2
2	3.5	2.5	0	0	70	2	0	13	2
1	2.5	2	0	0	75	2	0	14	1
2	3	1	0.5	0	23	0	4	33	0
2	1	0	0	0	210	0	4	24	<1
3	3.5	0.5	0.5	0	230	0	4	27	1
2	5	2	1	0	280	0	4	26	1
2	3.5	1	1	0	220	0	4	28	0
2	7	3	1	0	210	20	8	30	0
2	2	0.5	0.5	0	190	2	2	29	1
2	3.5	1	1	0	190	0	2	22	0

Muffins (box/pouch mixes) – Mustard FOOD NAME	Portion Size	Calories	
Triple Berry, Pouch	1/8 pkg	120	
Twice the Blueberries, mix	1/4 c	120	
Wild Blueberry	1/12 pkg	130	
Wild Blueberry low-fat	3 Tbs	110	
Bobs Red Mill			
Date Nut Bran, prep	1	70	
Oat Bran & Date Nut, prep	1	120	
Spice Apple Bran, prep	1	70	
Jiffy			
Apple Cinnamon, mix	1/4 c	160	
Banana Nut, mix	1/4 c	150	
Blueberry, mix	1/4 c	170	
Bran, mix	1/4 c	140	
Raspberry, mix	1/4 c	170	
MUSHROOMS			
B in B canned, slices	3 oz	30	
Brown or Italian, raw	1 oz	6	
Green Giant, canned, whole or slices	1/2 c	25	
Portobello, raw, diced	1 c	22	
Shiitake, cooked, no salt	1 c	81	
MUSSELS			
Blue, cooked	3 oz	146	
Gold Seal, in cottonseed oil, whole, smoked	2 oz	100	
MUSTARD			

Protein (g)	Total Fat (g)	Sat. Fat (g)	Trans Fat (g)	Chol. (mg)	Sodium (mg)	Calcium (%)	Iron (%)	Carbs (g)	Fiber (g)
2	3	1	0.5	15	220	0	4	22	0
2	1	0	0	0	180	0	2	26	1
2	1.5	0.5	0	0	210	0	2	27	<1
2	0	0	0	0	190	20	4	26	0
2	0.5	0	0	0	160	na	na	13	2
4	1.5	0	0	0	160	na	na	22	2
2	0	0	0	0	180	na	na	16	3
2	6	2	0	<5	300	4	4	25	0
2	6	2	0	<5	310	4	6	24	1
2	6	2.5	0.5	<5	310	4	6	26	0
2	4.5	1.5	0	<5	270	4	8	24	2
2	6	2.5	0.5	<5	310	4	6	26	0
2	1.5	0.5	0	5	460	0	0	3	0
1	0	0	0	0	2	1	1	1	0
2	0	0	0	0	440	0	2	4	1
2	0	0	0	0	5	1	3	4	1
2	0	0	0	0	6	0	4	21	3
20	4	1	0	48	314	3	32	6	0
13	4	1.5	0	45	150	4	90	2	0

FOOD NAME	Portion Size	Calories	
Grey Poupon, Country Dijon	1 tsp	5	
Grey Poupon, Honey Mustard	1 tsp	10	
Grey Poupon, Spicy Brown	1 tsp	5	
MUSTARD GREENS, cooked, chopped	1 c	21	
NECTARINE	2.5"	60	
NOODLES (dry)			
Light 'N Fluffy, Macaroni Dumpling	2 oz	210	
Light 'N Fluffy, medium	2 oz	210	
No Yolks	2 oz	210	
Pennsylvania Dutch, medium egg	1 c	220	
NOODLE DISHES (box mix); also see "Pasta"			
Lipton Asian Sides, Teriyaki, mix	⅔ c	240	
Lipton Pasta Sides, Alfredo, mix	⅔ c	240	
Lipton Pasta Sides, Beef, mix	⅔ c	210	
Lipton Pasta Sides, Butter, mix	⅔ c	240	
Lipton Pasta Sides, Cheddar Broccoli, mix	⅔ c	250	
Lipton Pasta Sides, Chicken, mix	⅔ c	220	
Lipton Pasta Sides, Stroganoff, mix	⅔ c	210	
OCEAN PERCH, Atlantic, broiled	3 oz	103	
OILS			
Avocado, Corn, Sesame, Soybean	1 Tbs	120	
Almond, Canola, Sunflower, Walnut	1 Tbs	120	
Mazola Right Blend (Corn & Canola)	1 Tbs	120	
OKRA, cooked, no salt, slices	½ c	18	
OLIVES			

Protein (g)	Total Fat (g)	Sat. Fat (g)	Trans Fat (g)	Chol. (mg)	Sodium (mg)	Calcium (%)	Iron (%)	Carbs (g)	Fiber (g)
0	0	0	0	0	120	0	0	0	0
0	0	0	0	0	5	0	0	2	0
0	0	0	0	0	50	0	0	0	0
3	0	0	0	0	22	10	5	3	3
1	0	0	0	0	0	1	2	14	2
7	1	0	0	0	0	na	10	42	2
8	2.5	1	0	15	40	na	10	40	2
8	0.5	0	0	0	30	na	na	41	3
8	3	1	0	65	15	2	10	40	2
7	2	0	0	0	780	2	15	49	2
8	4.5	2.5	0	10	810	8	10	40	1
7	1	0	0	0	830	2	10	43	1
7	4	2	0	10	780	2	10	43	1
10	3	1	0	<5	800	8	10	47	2
7	2	0	0	5	680	2	10	43	1
7	2	1	0	<5	780	2	10	39	1
20	2	0	0	46	82	12	6	0	0
0	14	2	0	0	0	0	0	0	0
0	14	1	0	0	0	0	0	0	0
0	14	1	0	0	0	0	0	0	0
1	0	0	0	0	5	6	1	4	2

FOOD NAME	Portion Size	Calories	
Lindsay, Black, large	4	25	
Lindsay, Green, medium	5	25	
Lindsay, Green, slices w/ Pimentos	2 Tbs	25	
Lindsay, Kalamata	3	25	
ONIONS			
Fresh, chopped, Yellow or Red	1 c	67	
Fresh, tops and bulbs (Scallions)	1 c	32	
Ore-Ida, frozen, Gourmet Rings	3 pcs	180	
Ore-Ida, frozen, Vidalia Os	4 pcs	180	
ORANGES			
Fresh, California	2-5/8"	59	
Fresh, Florida	2-5/8"	65	
Mandarin, canned (Dole)	½ c	80	
ORANGE JUICE/BEVERAGE			
Cascadian Farm, frozen, organic, prep	8 oz	110	
Dole, 100%	8 oz	120	
Dole, Orange, Peach, Mango	8 oz	120	
Minute Maid, country style	8 oz	110	
Minute Maid, home style & calcium & vitamin D	8 oz	110	
Minute Maid, Orange Passion	8 oz	130	
Minute Maid, Orange Tangerine	8 oz	110	
Tang, Orange, prep	8 oz	90	
Tang, Orange Pineapple, prep	8 oz	100	
Tang, Orange, sugar free, prep	8 oz	5	

Protein (g)	Total Fat (g)	Sat. Fat (g)	Trans Fat (g)	Chol. (mg)	Sodium (mg)	Calcium (%)	Iron (%)	Carbs (g)	Fiber (g)
0	2.5	0	0	0	115	na	na	1	0
0	2.5	0	0	0	115	na	na	1	0
0	2.5	0	0	0	330	na	na	<1	0
0	2.5	0	0	0	240	na	na	<1	0
1	0	0	0	0	5	4	2	16	2
2	0	0	0	0	15	7	8	7	3
3	8	1	0	0	320	0	4	25	1
2	10	1.5	0	0	280	0	6	22	1
1	0	0	0	0	0	5	1	14	3
1	0	0	0	0	0	6	5	16	3
0	0	0	0	0	10	0	2	19	1
1	0	0	0	0	0	na	na	27	0
<1	0	0	0	0	10	2	na	27	0
<1	0	0	0	0	10	2	na	28	0
2	0	0	0	0	15	2	na	27	0
2	0	0	0	0	15	35	na	27	0
1	0	0	0	0	20	35	na	31	0
2	0	0	0	0	15	35	na	27	0
0	0	0	0	0	35	10	0	23	0
0	0	0	0	0	45	6	0	24	0
0	0	0	0	0	0	2	0	0	0

FOOD NAME	Portion Size	Calories	
Tropicana, calcium & vitamin D	8 oz	110	
Tropicana, Essentials Light 'N Healthy	8 oz	50	
Tropicana, Essentials Fiber	8 oz	120	
Tropicana, original	8 oz	110	
OYSTERS			
Canned, smoked, in oil, can	3.75 oz	140	
Canned, whole	2 oz	80	
Eastern, raw	1 c	169	
Pacific, raw	3 oz	69	
PANCAKE/WAFFLE (mix)			
Aunt Jemima, Buckwheat, mix	¼ c	100	
Aunt Jemima, Buttermilk Complete, mix	⅓ c	160	
Aunt Jemima, original, mix	⅓ c	150	
Aunt Jemima, original complete, mix	⅓ c	160	
Aunt Jemima, Whole Wheat, mix	¼ c	120	
Bisquick Shake 'n Pour Buttermilk mix	½ c	200	
Hungry Jack, Buttermilk, mix	⅓ c	150	
Hungry Jack, Extra Light & Fluffy, mix	⅓ c	150	
Hungry Jack, original, mix	⅓ c	150	
Krusteaz, Blueberry, mix	½ c	240	
Krusteaz, Buttermilk, mix	½ c	210	
PANCAKE/WAFFLE (frozen)			
Aunt Jemima, Homestyle Waffles	2	190	
Aunt Jemima Magic Mini Pancakes, Cinnamon	13	240	

Protein (g)	Total Fat (g)	Sat. Fat (g)	Trans Fat (g)	Chol. (mg)	Sodium (mg)	Calcium (%)	Iron (%)	Carbs (g)	Fiber (g)
2	0	0	0	0	0	35	0	26	0
<1	0	0	0	0	10	20	0	13	0
2	0	0	0	0	0	2	0	29	3
2	0	0	0	0	0	2	0	26	0
10	8	2	0	45	280	2	30	8	0
7	3	1	0	35	220	2	30	6	0
17	6	2	0	131	523	11	92	10	0
8	2	0	0	43	90	1	24	4	0
4	1	0	0	0	580	4	10	23	3
5	2	0.5	0	10	460	15	10	31	1
4	0.5	0	0	0	740	10	10	33	1
5	1.5	0	0	5	470	15	10	32	1
4	0.5	0	0	0	620	6	15	26	3
6	3	0.5	0.5	0	730	8	8	39	1
4	1.5	0	0	<5	550	15	10	31	<1
4	2	0	0	<5	600	15	10	30	<1
4	1.5	0	0	0	550	15	10	31	<1
6	2.5	1	0	20	640	10	10	47	2
6	2	0.5	0	5	560	10	10	42	1
4	5	1	0	5	450	8	20	32	1
6	4	1	0	25	640	4	10	46	2

Pancake/Waffle (frozen) – Pancake Syrup FOOD NAME	Portion Size	Calories	
Aunt Jemima Magic Mini Pancakes, Strawberry	13	240	
Eggo, Apple Cinnamon, Blueberry, or Strawberry Waffles	2	190	
Eggo, Buttermilk Pancakes	3	280	
Eggo, Buttermilk Waffles	2	180	
Eggo, Chocolate Chip Waffles	2	200	
Eggo, Choco-'Nilla Flip-Flop Waffles	2	190	
Eggo, Special K Waffles	2	190	
Pillsbury			
Blueberry Pancakes	3	240	
Buttermilk Pancakes	3	240	
Chocolate Chip Pancakes	3	270	
Mini Blueberry Pancakes w/ Syrup	14	420	
Mini Buttermilk Pancakes w/ Syrup	14	410	
Original Pancakes	3	240	
Waffles, Blueberry	2	190	
Waffles, Buttermilk	2	170	
Waffles, Homestyle	2	170	
Waffle Sticks, Blueberry w/ Syrup	6	340	
Waffle Sticks, Chocolate Chip w/ Syrup	6	350	
Waffle Sticks, Cinnamon w/ Syrup	6	330	
PANCAKE SYRUP			
Aunt Jemima, butter lite	¼ c	100	
Aunt Jemima, butter rich	¼ c	210	

Protein (g)	Total Fat (g)	Sat. Fat (g)	Trans Fat (g)	Chol. (mg)	Sodium (mg)	Calcium (%)	Iron (%)	Carbs (g)	Fiber (g)
6	4	1	0	25	640	4	10	46	2
4	6	1.5	0	15	370	10	20	30	<1
6	9	1.5	0	15	580	4	20	44	1
5	6	1.5	2	15	420	10	20	26	1
4	6	1.5	2	15	380	10	20	32	1
4	7	1.5	2.5	15	360	10	20	28	1
15	11	2	2	0	350	20	20	15	7
5	4	1	1	10	440	10	10	46	2
6	4	1	1	10	470	10	10	47	2
6	5	2	1	10	430	10	10	50	2
4	7	1.5	1.5	5	520	6	10	86	<1
4	7	1.5	1.5	10	540	6	10	84	<1
5	4	1	1	10	640	6	10	46	1
3	5	1.5	1.5	0	480	0	20	32	<1
4	5	1.5	1.5	0	480	2	20	28	<1
3	5	1.5	1.5	0	540	2	20	29	<1
4	7	2	1.5	0	620	2	20	67	1
4	7	2	1.5	0	630	2	20	68	1
4	6	2	1.5	0	620	4	20	64	1
0	0	0	0	0	210	na	na	26	1
0	0	0	0	0	210	na	na	53	na

FOOD NAME	Portion Size	Calories	
Aunt Jemima, lite	¼ c	100	
Aunt Jemima, original	¼ c	210	
Log Cabin, sugar free	¼ c	35	
Maple Grove Farms	¼ c	200	
Vermont Maid	¼ c	210	
PALM, hearts, canned (Haddon House)	1.5 sticks	20	
PAPAYA			
Fresh, cubed	1 c	55	
Nectar (Knudsen)	8 oz	140	
Nectar, creamed	8 oz	40	
PARSNIPS, fresh, cooked, no salt	½ c	55	
PASTA—Bowls/Boxes			
Betty Crocker			
Bowl Appetit, Cheddar, Broccoli, Pasta	1 bowl	330	
Bowl Appetit, Chicken Pasta	1 bowl	260	
Bowl Appetit, Garlic Parmesan Pasta	1 bowl	320	
Bowl Appetit, Pasta Alfredo	1 bowl	360	
Bowl Appetit, Three-Cheese Rotini	1 bowl	360	
Chicken Helper, Cheddar & Broccoli, mix	½ c	160	
Chicken Helper, Chicken Fettuccine, mix	½ c	140	
Chicken Helper, Four Cheese, mix	⅔ c	160	
Cookbook Favorite Garlic & Herb			
Chicken Penne, mix	⅓ c	150	
Suddenly Pasta Salad, Caesar	½ c	170	
Suddenly Pasta Salad, Classic	⅔ c	180	

Protein (g)	Total Fat (g)	Sat. Fat (g)	Trans Fat (g)	Chol. (mg)	Sodium (mg)	Calcium (%)	Iron (%)	Carbs (g)	Fiber (g)
0	0	0	0	0	190	na	na	26	1
0	0	0	0	0	120	na	na	na	na
0	0	0	0	0	100	na	na	12	na
0	0	0	0	0	5	6	8	53	na
0	0	0	0	0	25	na	na	53	na
2	0	0	0	0	450	4	2	3	2
1	0	0	0	0	4	3	1	14	3
<1	0	0	0	0	35	2	0	35	0
<1	0	0	0	0	10	0	0	10	2
1	0	0	0	0	8	3	3	13	3
11	11	3.5	3	10	1000	10	15	49	2
9	6	2	1	10	790	2	8	42	2
11	9	3	2.5	10	1010	10	8	50	1
13	11	4	3.5	15	850	15	10	53	1
13	10	4	2.5	15	1020	15	10	55	2
5	4.5	1.5	1.5	5	690	4	6	24	1
4	3	1	1	0	700	0	4	25	1
5	5	2	1.5	5	670	4	4	24	1
5	5	1	0	0	380	4	8	21	2
6	1	0	0	0	650	2	8	34	1
6	1	0	0	0	860	4	10	37	2

Pasta—Bowls/Boxes

FOOD NAME	Portion Size	Calories	
Suddenly Pasta Salad, Creamy Italian	⅓ c	160	
Suddenly Pasta Salad, Ranch & Bacon	½ c	160	
Tuna Helper, Cheesy Pasta, mix	¾ c	150	
Tuna Helper, Creamy Broccoli, mix	½ c	190	
Tuna Helper, Creamy Parmesan, mix	¾ c	180	
Tuna Helper, Creamy Pasta, mix	¾ c	180	
Tuna Helper, Fettucinne Alfredo, mix	¾ c	170	
Canned			
Campbell's Beef Raviolio in Meat Sauce	1 c	270	
Campbell's Spaghetti in Tomato & Cheese	1 c	200	
SpaghettiOs	1 c	180	
SpaghettiOs, A to Z w/ Meatballs	1 c	260	
SpaghettiOs, A to Z, w/ Sliced Franks	1 c	230	
SpaghettiOs, w/ Meatballs	1 c	240	
SpaghettiOs Plus Calcium	1 c	170	
Dry			
Corn, Angel Hair (Westbrae)	2 oz	210	
Durum Wheat, various brands	2 oz	210	
Kamut, organic (Eden Foods)	2 oz	210	
Rye, organic (Eden Foods)	2 oz	200	
Spinach spaghetti (Westbrae)	2 oz	180	
Whole Wheat (DeCecco)	2 oz	180	
Whole Wheat Lasagna (Westbrae)	2 oz	180	
Whole Wheat Spaghetti (Westbrae)	2 oz	200	
Refrigerated—Buitoni			

Protein (g)	Total Fat (g)	Sat. Fat (g)	Trans Fat (g)	Chol. (mg)	Sodium (mg)	Calcium (%)	Iron (%)	Carbs (g)	Fiber (g)
7	1.5	0.5	0	0	450	4	8	32	2
7	1.5	0	0	0	360	2	8	31	1
5	1.5	0.5	0.5	<5	750	2	4	30	1
6	5	1.5	na	0	680	0	6	31	1
6	2.5	0.5	1	0	890	2	6	33	2
5	5	1.5	2	0	730	0	4	30	1
5	3	1	1	0	830	2	6	30	1
11	8	3.5	0	20	1090	4	10	38	4
7	1.5	0.5	0	5	950	2	4	40	3
6	1	0.5	0	5	850	2	10	37	3
11	9	3.5	0	20	990	15	15	33	3
9	7	2.5	0	15	990	15	15	33	2
11	8	3.5	0	25	890	15	20	32	3
6	1	0.5	0	5	620	30	10	35	3
4	1.5	0	0	0	15	0	2	46	0
7	1	0	0	0	0	na	10	42	2
10	1.5	0.5	0	0	0	2	15	38	6
6	0	0	0	0	10	2	10	44	8
9	2	0	0	0	20	2	15	38	8
8	1.5	0	0	<5	0	2	10	35	7
8	1.5	0	0	0	5	0	8	34	7
9	1.5	0	0	0	10	0	10	39	9

FOOD NAME	Portion Size	Calories	
Angel Hair Pasta	1¼ c	230	
Linguine	1¼ c	240	
Ravioli, Classic Beef	1¼ c	350	
Ravioli, Four Cheese	1⅓ c	330	
Ravioli, Garden Vegetable	1 c	250	
Tortellini, Cheese & Roasted Garlic	1 c	270	
Tortellini, Mozzarella & Pepperoni	1 c	330	
Tortellini, Spinach Cheese	1 c	320	
Tortellini, Sweet Italian Sausage	1 c	330	
Tortellini, Three Cheese	1 c	330	
PASTA SAUCE			
Buitoni			
Alfredo	½ c	140	
Light	½ c	80	
Marinara	½ c	70	
Pesto w/ Basil	¼ c	300	
Tomato Herb Parmesan	½ c	130	
Classico			
Alfredo	¼ c	120	
Basil Pesto	¼ c	230	
Florentine Spinach & Cheese	½ c	80	
Italian Sausage w/ Pepper & Onion	½ c	90	
Roasted Garlic	½ c	60	
Tomato & Basil	½ c	60	
Del Monte			

Protein (g)	Total Fat (g)	Sat. Fat (g)	Trans Fat (g)	Chol. (mg)	Sodium (mg)	Calcium (%)	Iron (%)	Carbs (g)	Fiber (g)
10	2.5	1	0	45	20	2	10	43	2
10	2.5	1	0	50	20	2	10	45	2
15	11	3.5	0	60	540	6	15	47	2
14	10	6	0	60	550	15	10	45	3
11	5	2	0	50	480	10	6	40	2
12	8	4	0	35	360	15	6	38	2
15	10	4.5	0	45	510	15	10	45	3
15	7	3.5	0	55	510	20	10	49	3
13	10	3	0	35	300	4	10	48	3
15	8	3.5	0	40	480	15	10	50	3
4	11	7	0	35	430	10	0	5	0
4	5	3.5	0	15	360	10	0	5	0
1	3	0.5	0	0	580	6	2	10	2
7	28	5	0	20	540	15	10	6	2
4	8	2.5	0	10	750	10	4	10	2
2	2	0	0	0	340	4	6	11	2
3	21	3	0	0	720	6	4	6	1
3	5	1	0	.5	560	6	2	6	2
5	2	1	0	5	470	6	10	13	2
2	1	0	0	0	220	6	8	11	2
2	1	0	0	0	310	6	8	11	2

Pasta Sauce FOOD NAME	Portion Size	Calories	
Italian Herb Chunky	½ c	60	
Spaghetti Sauce w/ Four Cheeses	½ c	70	
Spaghetti Sauce w/ Meat	½ c	60	
Spaghetti Sauce w/ Mushrooms	½ c	60	
DiGiorno Microwaveable			
Alfredo	2.5 oz	180	
Alfredo, Four Cheese	2.5 oz	160	
Alfredo, reduced fat	2.5 oz	130	
Basil Pesto	2.3 oz	310	
Marinara	3.5 oz	70	
Eden Foods			
Pizza Pasta Sauce, organic	½ c	65	
Spaghetti Sauce, organic	½ c	80	
Hunt's			
Four Cheese	½ c	50	
Meat	½ c	60	
Mushroom	½ c	45	
Muir Glen Organic			
Fire Roasted Tomato	½ c	70	
Four Cheese	½ c	80	
Garden Vegetable	½ c	60	
Mushroom Marinara	½ c	50	
Tomato Basil	½ c	60	
Newman's Own			
Bombolina	½ c	90	

Protein (g)	Total Fat (g)	Sat. Fat (g)	Trans Fat (g)	Chol. (mg)	Sodium (mg)	Calcium (%)	Iron (%)	Carbs (g)	Fiber (g)
2	1	0	0	0	520	4	6	12	<1
2	1.5	0	0	0	680	4	4	15	3
3	1	0	0	2	720	4	8	14	3
2	0.5	0	0	0	630	4	8	14	2
3	17	3	0	15	720	8	0	3	0
5	15	6	0	30	700	15	0	3	0
4	8	5	0	30	910	15	0	10	0
6	31	4.5	0.5	15	530	20	2	2	1
2	1.5	0	0	0	230	4	6	12	2
2	2.5	0	0	0	300	4	10	9	5
3	2.5	0	0	0	320	8	6	12	3
3	1	0	0	0	580	4	20	10	3
3	1	0	0	0	610	2	10	11	3
2	0.5	0	0	0	500	2	10	10	3
2	2	0	0	0	340	4	6	11	2
4	3	1	0	5	380	6	8	11	2
2	1	0	0	0	350	2	6	10	2
2	0	0	0	0	340	2	8	10	2
2	1	0	0	0	370	2	8	12	2
2	4.5	0.5	0	0	620	2	8	13	<1

FOOD NAME	Portion Size	Calories	
Five Cheese	½ c	80	
Italian Sausage & Pepper	½ c	90	
Marinara	½ c	70	
Pesto & Tomato	½ c	60	
Vodka Sauce	½ c	110	
Prego			
Chunky Garden, Mushroom Supreme	½ c	120	
Chunky Garden, Tomato, Onion & Garlic	½ c	110	
Fresh Mushroom	½ c	120	
Hearty Meat, Three Meat Supreme	½ c	170	
Italian Sausage & Garlic	½ c	120	
Organic Mushroom	½ c	90	
Roasted Garlic Parmesan	½ c	100	
Progresso			
Lobster	½ c	100	
Red Clam	½ c	60	
White Clam	½ c	130	
Ragu			
Chunky, Sundried Tomato & Basil	½ c	120	
Chunky Super Vegetable Primavera	½ c	110	
Light, Tomato & Basil	½ c	60	
Organic Cheese	½ c	80	
Robusto, Parmesan & Romano	½ c	90	
PASTRAMI			
Beef, 98% f-f	2 oz	54	

Protein (g)	Total Fat (g)	Sat. Fat (g)	Trans Fat (g)	Chol. (mg)	Sodium (mg)	Calcium (%)	Iron (%)	Carbs (g)	Fiber (g)
3	3	1.5	0	5	610	0	4	10	<1
4	4	1	0	10	630	4	6	11	<1
2	2	0	0	0	510	4	10	12	<1
2	1	0	0	0	310	6	8	11	2
5	5	1.5	0	5	440	na	na	11	0
2	4	1	0	0	500	2	4	19	4
2	3.5	0.5	0	0	520	2	4	17	0
2	3.5	1	0	0	570	2	4	18	3
7	10	4	0	15	650	2	4	13	3
3	5	1.5	0	10	500	2	4	16	3
2	2.5	0	0	0	540	2	4	13	4
3	1	0.5	0	5	550	4	4	20	3
3	7	1	0	5	430	2	6	6	2
4	1	0	0	10	350	2	4	8	1
6	10	1.5	0	10	750	2	8	5	0
2	3	0	0	0	510	4	6	21	2
2	3	0	0	18	490	4	6	18	3
2	0	0	0	0	360	4	6	12	2
2	3	0.5	0	0	490	4	6	11	2
3	3	0.5	0	<5	590	6	6	12	2
11	1	0	0	27	576	1	9	1	0

FOOD NAME	Portion Size	Calories	
Carl Buddig, beef, chopped, pressed	2 oz	80	
Sara Lee beef, pre-sliced	2 slices	60	
PASTRY—Toaster			
Kellogg's Pop-Tarts			
Apple Cinnamon	1	210	
Blueberry	1	210	
Chocolate Chip Cookie Dough	1	200	
French Toast	1	220	
Frosted Cherry	1	200	
Frosted Chocolate Fudge	1	200	
Frosted Cookies & Crème	1	200	
Frosted Raspberry	1	210	
Frosted S'mores	1	200	
Low-fat Frosted Brown Sugar Cinnamon	1	190	
Low-fat Frosted Chocolate Fudge	1	190	
Pillsbury Toaster Strudel			
Apple	1	190	
Blueberry	1	190	
Brown Sugar Cinnamon	1	200	
Chocolate Fudge	1	210	
Cream Cheese	1	200	
Cream Cheese & Raspberry	1	200	
S'mores	1	200	
Strawberry	1	190	
Wild Berry	1	190	

Protein (g)	Total Fat (g)	Sat. Fat (g)	Trans Fat (g)	Chol. (mg)	Sodium (mg)	Calcium (%)	Iron (%)	Carbs (g)	Fiber (g)
11	4	2	0	37	602	1	8	1	0
9	2.5	1	0	25	380	0	8	0	0
2	6	3	0	0	180	0	10	37	<1
2	6	3	0	0	180	0	10	37	<1
2	5	2.5	0	0	190	0	10	35	<1
3	8	4	0	0	180	0	10	35	<1
2	5	2.5	0	0	210	2	10	37	<1
3	5	2.5	0	0	210	2	10	37	<1
3	5	2.5	0	0	260	0	10	35	<1
2	5	2.5	0	0	160	0	10	38	<1
3	5	2.5	0	0	210	0	10	36	<1
3	3	1.5	0	0	210	0	10	38	<1
2	3	1.5	0	0	260	0	10	38	<1
2	9	3.5	1	5	190	10	10	25	<1
3	9	3.5	1	5	190	10	10	26	<1
3	9	3.5	1	5	220	10	10	28	1
3	10	4	1.5	5	220	10	10	26	<1
3	11	4.5	1.5	10	220	10	10	23	0
3	10	4	1	10	210	10	10	24	0
3	9	3.5	1	5	200	10	10	27	<1
3	9	3.5	1	5	190	10	10	25	<1
3	9	3.5	1	5	190	10	10	25	<1

FOOD NAME	Portion Size	Calories	
PEACHES, fresh, raw	2.5"	38	
Canned			
Del Monte, Carb Clever, sliced	½ c	30	
Del Monte, Freestone Slices	½ c	100	
Del Monte Fruit Naturals, chunks	½ c	70	
Del Monte Harvest Spice, sliced	½ c	80	
S&W, halves	½ c	70	
S&W, natural style	½ c	80	
S&W Snow Peaches	½ c	80	
Dried, sulfured, halves	1 c	382	
Frozen, Cascadian Farm, sliced, organic	1 c	60	
Juice/nectar			
Knudsen	8 oz	130	
Santa Cruz, organic	8 oz	120	
PEANUT BUTTER			
Jif, creamy	2 Tbs	190	
Jif, creamy & honey	2 Tbs	190	
Jif, reduced fat	2 Tbs	190	
Maranatha Organic, creamy	2 Tbs	190	
Maranatha Organic, crunch	2 Tbs	190	
Peter Pan, creamy	2 Tbs	190	
Skippy, honey roasted creamy	2 Tbs	190	
Skippy, reduced fat, creamy	2 Tbs	190	
Skippy, regular creamy	2 Tbs	190	
Skippy, super chunk	2 Tbs	190	

Protein (g)	Total Fat (g)	Sat. Fat (g)	Trans Fat (g)	Chol. (mg)	Sodium (mg)	Calcium (%)	Iron (%)	Carbs (g)	Fiber (g)
1	0	0	0	0	0	1	1	9	1
1	0	0	0	0	10	0	3	7	1
0	0	0	0	0	10	0	0	24	1
<1	0	0	0	0	10	0	0	17	<1
<1	0	0	0	0	10	0	0	21	<1
0	0	0	0	0	10	0	0	17	1
1	0	0	0	0	20	0	0	19	1
<1	0	0	0	0	15	0	0	20	1
6	1	0	0	0	11	4	36	98	13
1	0	0	0	0	0	0	2	14	1
1	0	0	0	0	15	2	4	31	0
1	0	0	0	0	10	na	na	29	0
8	16	3	0	0	150	0	4	7	2
6	15	2.5	0	0	120	0	4	11	2
8	12	2.5	0	0	250	0	4	15	2
8	16	2.5	0	0	80	2	4	7	2
8	16	2.5	0	0	80	2	4	7	2
7	17	3.5	0	0	140	0	2	6	2
7	17	3.5	0	0	125	0	2	7	2
7	12	2.5	0	0	190	0	4	15	2
7	16	3	0	0	150	0	4	7	2
7	17	3.5	0	0	140	0	2	7	2

FOOD NAME	Portion Size	Calories	
Peanut Butter – Peas, fresh, boiled, no salt			
Smart Balance Omega, creamy	2 Tbs	190	
Smucker's natural, creamy or chunky	2 Tbs	210	
Smucker's natural, reduced fat creamy	2 Tbs	200	
PEANUTS			
Dry Roasted, w/ salt	1 oz	165	
Oil Roasted, w/ salt	1 oz	169	
Planters, Honey roasted	1 oz	160	
Planters, Sweet n' Crunchy	1 oz	140	
PEARS, fresh, raw	1 med	96	
Canned/jarred			
Del Monte, Bartlett, Cinnamon halves	½ c	80	
Del Monte, Bartlett, halves, light syrup	½ c	60	
Del Monte, Bartlett, Orchard Select	½ c	80	
S&W, Bartlett, halves, light syrup	½ c	80	
S&W, Bartlett, slices, natural style	½ c	80	
Nectar, Santa Cruz, organic	8 oz	120	
PEAS, fresh, boiled, no salt	1 c	134	
Canned			
Del Monte, Peas & Carrots	½ c	60	
Del Monte, Sweet Peas	½ c	60	
Del Monte, Very Young Small Sweet	½ c	60	
Green Giant, LeSueur Early Peas	⅔ c	60	
Stokely, Peas & Pearl Onions	½ c	40	
Frozen			
Green Giant, Baby Sweet Peas & Butter	¾ c	90	

Protein (g)	Total Fat (g)	Sat. Fat (g)	Trans Fat (g)	Chol. (mg)	Sodium (mg)	Calcium (%)	Iron (%)	Carbs (g)	Fiber (g)
7	16	2.5	0	0	110	0	4	6	2
8	16	2.5	0	0	120	0	2	6	2
9	12	2	0	0	120	0	2	12	2
7	14	2	0	0	230	2	4	6	2
8	15	2	0	0	90	2	2	4	3
6	13	1.5	0	0	95	0	4	8	2
4	7	1	0	0	20	0	2	16	2
<1	0	0	0	0	2	1	2	26	5
0	0	0	0	0	10	0	0	21	1
0	0	0	0	0	10	0	0	15	1
<1	0	0	0	0	10	0	0	20	2
0	0	0	0	0	10	0	0	19	2
0	0	0	0	0	10	0	2	21	2
0	0	0	0	0	30	4	2	30	0
9	0	0	0	0	5	4	14	25	9
2	0	0	0	0	360	2	4	11	2
3	0	0	0	0	390	2	8	13	4
3	0	0	0	0	360	0	8	10	4
4	0	0	0	0	380	2	6	12	3
3	0	0	0	0	530	0	6	10	3
5	1.5	0.5	0	<5	410	0	6	14	4

Peas, fresh, boiled, no salt – Pickles FOOD NAME	Portion Size	Calories	
Green Giant, Select Early June Peas	⅔ c	60	
Green Giant, Sugar Snap Peas	½ c	40	
Green Giant, Sweet w/Tiny Pearl Onions	½ c	60	
PECANS			
Planters, Chips	2 oz	390	
Planters, fresh, unsalted halves	1 oz	190	
PEPPERS			
Bruno, Banana Wax Peppers	4 pcs	10	
Bruno, Mild Wax Peppers	11 pcs	8	
Fresh, raw, Green, chopped	1 c	30	
Fresh, raw, Red, chopped	1 c	39	
Fresh, raw, Yellow, large	3"	50	
Vlasic, Pepper Rings	12	5	
Vlasic, Zesty Cherry Peppers	2	10	
PEPPERONI			
Hormel, original	14 slices	140	
Smart Deli, slices (soy)	13 slices	45	
PICKLES			
Cascadian Farms, Baby Dills	1⅓ pcs	5	
Cascadian Farms, Bread & Butter chips	5	30	
Claussen Bread 'n Butter, Sandwich Slices	1 oz	5	
Claussen Half Sours, New York deli style	1 oz	5	
Claussen Kosher Dill Halves	1 oz	5	
Claussen Kosher Dill Spears	1 oz	5	
Claussen Kosher Dill Burger Slices	1 oz	5	

Protein (g)	Total Fat (g)	Sat. Fat (g)	Trans Fat (g)	Chol. (mg)	Sodium (mg)	Calcium (%)	Iron (%)	Carbs (g)	Fiber (g)
4	0.5	0	0	0	150	0	4	11	4
2	0	0	0	0	95	4	4	10	2
4	0	0	0	0	440	0	4	11	3
5	40	3	0	0	5	4	8	9	7
3	20	1.5	0	0	0	2	4	4	3
0	0	0	0	0	280	na	na	1	0
0	0	0	0	0	260	na	na	1	0
1	0	0	0	0	4	1	3	7	3
1	0	0	0	0	3	1	4	9	3
2	0	0	0	0	4	2	5	12	2
0	0	0	0	0	480	0	0	1	0
0	0	0	0	0	480	0	0	1	0
5	13	6	0	35	490	0	2	0	0
8	0	0	0	0	300	na	na	3	1
0	0	0	0	0	300	0	0	1	0
0	0	0	0	0	110	0	0	8	0
3	0	0	0	0	210	0	0	5	0
0	0	0	0	0	260	0	0	1	0
0	0	0	0	0	330	0	0	1	0
0	0	0	0	0	330	0	0	1	0
0	0	0	0	0	300	0	0	1	0

Pickles – Pie Filling / FOOD NAME	Portion Size	Calories	
Claussen Sweet Gerkins	1 oz	30	
Del Monte, sweet, midget	1 oz	40	
Del Monte, sweet, whole	1 oz	40	
PIES—Frozen			
Edward's Chocolate Butter Pecan	1 pc	560	
Edward's Chocolate Cream	⅛ pie	450	
Edward's Georgia Pecan	⅛ pie	490	
Edward's Key Lime	⅛ pie	450	
Edward's Oreo Cream	⅛ pie	480	
Edward's Turtle	⅛ pie	390	
Marie Callender, Apple	⅒ pie	350	
Marie Callender's, Pumpkin	⅛ pie	330	
Mrs. Smith's, Blueberry	⅛ pie	330	
Mrs. Smith's, Cherry	⅛ pie	330	
Mrs. Smith, 'Coconut Custard	⅛ pie	290	
Mrs. Smith's, Sweet Potato	⅛ pie	350	
Sara Lee, Apple	⅛ pie	340	
Sara Lee, Blueberry	⅛ pie	350	
Sara Lee, Dutch Apple	⅛ pie	340	
PIECRUST			
Pet-Ritz, deep dish	⅛ pie	90	
Pet-Ritz, deep dish, all vegetable	⅛ pie	90	
Pet-Ritz, regular	⅛ pie	80	
Pillsbury all ready rolled	⅛ pie	120	
PIE FILLING			

Protein (g)	Total Fat (g)	Sat. Fat (g)	Trans Fat (g)	Chol. (mg)	Sodium (mg)	Calcium (%)	Iron (%)	Carbs (g)	Fiber (g)
0	0	0	0	0	210	0	0	7	0
0	0	0	0	0	210	0	0	10	<1
0	0	0	0	0	210	0	0	10	<1
5	32	14	na	90	270	2	10	63	2
5	27	15	3.5	15	320	8	10	48	1
5	26	4.5	3.5	75	280	0	6	60	1
6	22	15	1.5	50	310	20	4	58	0
4	30	17	3.5	0	320	6	10	50	1
4	22	11	2.5	10	270	6	6	46	1
2	19	4.5	5	0	170	0	6	42	1
6	14	3	3	35	220	15	8	46	2
3	16	7	0	0	370	0	4	44	2
3	16	7	0	0	280	0	4	44	1
7	16	6	2.5	60	310	10	4	31	<1
4	18	7	0	40	210	4	6	44	1
3	15	7	0	0	340	0	8	51	2
3	15	7	0	0	340	0	8	51	2
3	14	6	0	0	290	0	8	52	2
1	5	2	0	<5	85	0	4	11	0
1	5	1	1.5	0	85	0	4	11	0
1	4	1.5	0	0	70	0	2	9	0
<1	7	2.5	0	<5	110	0	0	13	0

FOOD NAME	Portion Size	Calories	
Pie Filling – Pineapple, fresh, diced			
Comstock			
Apple	½ c	30	
Blueberry, more fruit	½ c	100	
Cherry, more fruit	½ c	100	
Lucky Leaf			
Apple	⅓ c	90	
Apricot	⅓ c	90	
Blueberry, premium	⅓ c	100	
Coconut Crème	⅓ c	100	
Lemon Cream	⅓ c	130	
Pineapple	⅓ c	100	
Raisin	⅓ c	90	
Strawberry, premium	½ c	100	
PIEROGIES			
Mrs. T's, American Cheese	3	210	
Mrs. T's, Broccoli & Cheddar	3	200	
Mrs. T's, Four Cheese	3	230	
Mrs. T's, Sour Cream	3	210	
PINEAPPLE, fresh, diced	1 c	74	
Del Monte, chunks in heavy syrup	½ c	90	
Del Monte, chunks in own juice	½ c	70	
Del Monte, crushed, heavy syrup	½ c	90	
Del Monte, Fruit Naturals	½ c	70	
Dole, fruit bowl	4 oz	60	
Dole, fruit bowl in lime gel	4.3 oz	90	

Protein (g)	Total Fat (g)	Sat. Fat (g)	Trans Fat (g)	Chol. (mg)	Sodium (mg)	Calcium (%)	Iron (%)	Carbs (g)	Fiber (g)
0	0	0	0	0	10	0	0	7	2
0	0	0	0	0	25	0	2	23	1
0	0	0	0	0	15	0	0	23	1
0	0	0	0	0	40	0	0	22	2
0	0	0	0	0	55	0	2	22	0
0	0	0	0	0	45	0	0	24	1
1	2	0	0	0	140	0	2	25	3
0	1	0	0	10	220	0	4	31	0
0	0	0	0	0	35	0	2	23	1
0	0	0	0	0	75	0	4	22	0
0	0	0	0	0	25	0	2	23	1
8	6	3	0	15	570	8	8	32	1
6	4.5	1	1	5	560	4	10	33	2
6	7	1.5	0	10	570	4	8	36	1
6	5	2	0.5	15	510	4	10	34	1
1	0	0	0	0	2	2	2	20	2
0	0	0	0	0	10	0	2	24	1
0	0	0	0	0	10	0	2	17	1
0	0	0	0	0	10	0	2	24	1
<1	0	0	0	0	5	0	0	18	<1
<1	0	0	0	0	10	0	0	16	1
<1	0	0	0	0	95	0	0	23	0

FOOD NAME	Portion Size	Calories	
Dole, slices in 100% juice	2 pcs	60	
Dole, tidbits in 100% juice	½ c	60	
PINEAPPLE JUICE/BEVERAGE			
Dole 100%	8 oz	120	
Dole, Pineapple Orange, 100%	6 oz	100	
Knudsen, nectar	8 oz	140	
Knudsen, Pineapple Coconut	8 oz	130	
Santa Cruz, Orange Pineapple	8 oz	100	
Santa Cruz, Pineapple Coconut	8 oz	130	
PISTACHIOS, dry roasted (Planters)	1 oz	170	
PIZZA (frozen); also see "Fast Food"			
Amy's Kitchen			
Cheese	⅓ pie	310	
Mediterranean w/ Cornmeal Crust	⅓ pie	360	
Pesto	⅓ pie	310	
Rice Crust, Cheese	⅓ pie	300	
Roasted Vegetable	⅓ pie	270	
Soy Cheese	⅓ pie	290	
Three Cheese w/ cornmeal crust	⅓ pie	370	
DiGiorno			
Cheese Stuffed Crust	⅙ pie	350	
Cheese Stuffed Crust, Three meat	⅙ pie	340	
Cheese Stuffed Crust, Pepperoni	⅕ pie	370	
Cheese Stuffed Crust, Four cheese	⅕ pie	360	
Deep Dish, Three Meat	⅙ pie	310	

Protein (g)	Total Fat (g)	Sat. Fat (g)	Trans Fat (g)	Chol. (mg)	Sodium (mg)	Calcium (%)	Iron (%)	Carbs (g)	Fiber (g)
0	0	0	0	0	10	0	2	15	1
0	0	0	0	0	10	0	2	15	1
1	0	0	0	0	10	2	4	29	0
0	0	0	0	0	na	2	0	24	0
1	0	0	0	0	20	2	2	35	0
1	1	0.5	0	0	50	4	2	31	0
0	0	0	0	0	0	2	0	24	0
1	1	0.5	0.5	0	20	2	4	30	0
5	14	2	0	0	190	2	6	0	3
12	12	4	0	15	590	20	4	38	2
12	15	4.5	0	15	680	20	10	45	3
12	12	3.5	0	10	480	15	15	39	2
11	14	4	0	15	590	20	10	31	2
6	9	1.5	0	0	490	2	4	42	2
12	11	1	0	0	590	2	10	37	2
10	19	4	0	10	580	10	15	41	2
18	15	7	0	35	950	2	8	35	3
17	16	7	0.5	35	940	20	8	34	2
19	16	8	0.5	40	1030	25	10	40	3
19	14	8	0.5	35	940	30	8	41	3
13	15	6	1.5	25	790	15	6	32	2

Pizza (frozen)		
FOOD NAME	Portion Size	Calories
Deep Dish, Pepperoni	⅙ pie	340
Deep Dish, Supreme	⅙ pie	320
Microwave Rising Crust, Pepperoni	½ pie	390
Microwave Rising Crust, Supreme	½ pie	400
Thin Crispy Crust, Four Meat	⅕ pie	320
Thin Crispy Crust, Harvest Wheat Supreme	⅕ pie	250
Thin Crispy Crust, Harvest Wheat Pepperoni	⅕ pie	270
Thin Crispy Crust, Supreme	⅕ pie	300
Jeno's Crisp'n Tasty		
Canadian Bacon	1 pie	420
Cheese	1 pie	440
Combination	1 pie	490
Hamburger	1 pie	480
Pepperoni	1 pie	490
Sausage	1 pie	480
Supreme	1 pie	490
Three Meat	1 pie	480
Lean Cuisine		
Cheese French Bread	1 pkg	320
Delux French Bread	1 pkg	310
Pepperoni French Bread	1 pkg	300
Tombstone		
Brickoven Pepperoni	¼ pie	310

Protein (g)	Total Fat (g)	Sat. Fat (g)	Trans Fat (g)	Chol. (mg)	Sodium (mg)	Calcium (%)	Iron (%)	Carbs (g)	Fiber (g)
14	18	7	1.5	35	920	20	6	32	2
14	15	6	1.5	30	810	15	6	33	2
16	18	7	1.5	20	830	15	10	44	3
16	18	7	1.5	25	860	15	10	45	4
13	13	5	0	35	830	15	6	37	2
14	8	3.5	0	20	520	20	10	32	4
16	9	4	0	25	610	25	10	32	4
14	12	5	0	30	740	15	4	36	3
16	18	3.5	4.5	15	1150	15	15	49	2
16	21	5	5	15	1060	30	15	47	2
17	25	6	4.5	20	1160	15	15	50	2
21	22	5	4.5	25	1120	15	20	50	2
16	26	6	5	20	1170	15	15	50	2
16	24	6	4.5	20	1130	15	15	50	2
17	25	6	4.5	20	1150	15	15	49	2
17	24	6	4.5	20	1200	15	15	49	2
18	7	4	0	20	520	30	8	47	3
16	9	3.5	0	20	700	15	15	44	3
16	7	2.5	0	15	560	10	10	44	2
14	16	7	0	35	740	20	6	29	2

Pizza – Pizza Snacks FOOD NAME	Portion Size	Calories	
Brickoven Pepperoni & Sausage	¼ pie	320	
Brickoven, Supreme	¼ pie	320	
Double Top Pepperoni	⅕ pie	400	
Harvest Wheat Thin Crust, Cheese	⅓ pie	300	
Harvest Wheat Thin Crust, Supreme	¼ pie	260	
Light Veggie	⅕ pie	230	
Original, Extra Cheese	¼ pie	350	
Original, Sausage	⅕ pie	290	
Original, Supreme	⅕ pie	300	
Original, Four Meat	⅕ pie	310	
Totino's Party Pizza			
Canadian Bacon	½ pie	320	
Cheese	½ pie	320	
Combination	½ pie	380	
Hamburger	½ pie	360	
Mexican	½ pie	370	
Mini Meatball	½ pie	350	
Pepperoni	½ pie	360	
Sausage	½ pie	360	
Supreme	½ pie	360	
Three Cheese	½ pie	330	
Three Meat	½ pie	350	
PIZZA SNACKS			
Totino's Mexican Style, Chicken Fajita	6	190	
Totino's Mexican Style, Chicken & Cheese	6	190	

Protein (g)	Total Fat (g)	Sat. Fat (g)	Trans Fat (g)	Chol. (mg)	Sodium (mg)	Calcium (%)	Iron (%)	Carbs (g)	Fiber (g)
15	16	7	0	40	740	20	6	30	3
14	16	7	0	35	720	20	6	30	3
20	22	10	0.5	55	950	35	8	31	4
17	10	5	0	25	620	30	6	37	4
15	10	4.5	0	25	600	20	6	29	3
13	6	2	0	10	510	20	10	31	4
18	15	8	0.5	40	660	35	8	37	4
14	13	5	0	30	590	20	8	30	3
14	14	6	0	30	640	20	8	31	3
15	14	6	0	35	690	20	10	30	3
13	15	3	4	10	910	15	10	34	1
12	15	3.5	3.5	10	760	20	10	34	1
14	21	5	4	15	940	15	10	34	1
15	19	4.5	4.5	20	800	15	10	35	1
16	19	4.5	4.5	20	770	15	15	34	2
13	18	4	4	10	790	15	10	34	1
12	20	5	4	10	870	15	10	33	3
14	19	4	4	15	810	15	10	34	1
14	19	4.5	4	15	840	15	10	34	1
13	16	6	1.5	25	720	25	10	33	1
13	18	4	41	15	870	15	10	34	1
8	6	1.5	1.5	10	530	2	8	25	1
8	7	2	1	15	420	6	8	24	1

FOOD NAME	Portion Size	Calories
Totino's Pizza Rolls, Cheese	6	190
Totino's Pizza Rolls, Cheesy Taco	6	210
Totino's Pizza Rolls, Combination	6	220
Totino's Pizza Rolls, Pepperoni	6	210
Totino's Pizza Rolls, Sausage	6	210
Totino's Pizza Rolls, Supreme	6	210
Totino's Pizza Rolls, Three Meat	6	210
PLANTAIN, raw	1 c	181
PLUMS, raw	2⅛"	30
Canned, purple, light syrup	1 c	159
POMEGRANATE		
Fresh	½ fruit	80
Juice		
Knudsen, Just Pomegranate	8 oz	150
Knudsen, Vita Pomegranate	8 oz	130
POM, 100%	8 oz	160
POPCORN		
Air-Popped, plain, no salt	1 c	31
Healthy Choice, microwave,		
Butter, kernels	3 Tbs	120
Healthy Choice, microwave,		
Natural, kernels	3 Tbs	120
Jolly Time, microwave, Healthy Pop, kernel	2 Tbs	90
Jolly Time, microwave, Sassy		
Salsa, kernels	2 Tbs	180

Protein (g)	Total Fat (g)	Sat. Fat (g)	Trans Fat (g)	Chol. (mg)	Sodium (mg)	Calcium (%)	Iron (%)	Carbs (g)	Fiber (g)
8	6	1.5	1.5	5	480	10	8	26	1
7	10	4	1	20	440	8	6	23	1
8	11	3	1.5	10	470	4	8	24	1
8	10	2.5	1.5	10	480	4	10	25	1
8	10	2.5	1.5	10	410	4	8	24	1
7	9	2	1.5	10	390	4	8	25	2
8	9	2.5	1.5	10	470	4	8	24	1
2	1	0	0	0	6	0	5	47	3
0	0	0	0	0	0	0	1	8	1
1	0	0	0	0	50	2	12	41	2
1	0.5	0	0	0	27	2	6	18	<1
<1	0	0	0	0	20	0	6	38	0
0	0	0	0	0	10	15	0	33	0
0	0	0	0	0	10	0	0	40	0
1	0	0	0	0	0	0	1	6	1
4	3	0	0	0	330	2	4	25	5
4	2.5	0	0	0	330	2	4	26	5
3	2	0	0	0	210	0	4	23	9
2	13	3	6	0	400	0	4	16	4

FOOD NAME	Portion Size	Calories	
Jolly Time, microwave, Mallow Magic, kernels	2 Tbs	180	
Orville Redenbacher, Butter, kernels	3 Tbs	170	
Orville Redenbacher, Movie Theater, kernels	3 Tbs	170	
Orville Redenbacher, Smart Pop, kernels	3 Tbs	130	
Orville Redenbacher, Tender White, kernels	3 Tbs	180	
Wise, bagged, Butter Flavored	1 oz	150	
Wise, bagged, Hot Cheese	1 oz	150	
Wise, bagged, Lite Butter Flavored	1 oz	140	
PORK			
Fresh, center loin chops, lean & fat, broiled	3 oz	204	
Fresh, center rib chops, lean & fat, broiled	3 oz	224	
Fresh, center rib roast, lean, roasted	3 oz	182	
Fresh, loin blade chops, lean & fat, broiled	3 oz	272	
Fresh, spare ribs, braised, lean & fat	3 oz	337	
Fresh, tenderloin, lean, roasted	3 oz	139	
Fresh, tenderloin, lean & fat, roasted	3 oz	147	
Hormel Always Tender, boneless loin	4 oz	162	
Hormel Always Tender, center chops	4 oz	187	
PORK RINDS			
Wise, Hot & Spicy, BBQ	.625 oz	90	
Wise, original	.625 oz	90	

Protein (g)	Total Fat (g)	Sat. Fat (g)	Trans Fat (g)	Chol. (mg)	Sodium (mg)	Calcium (%)	Iron (%)	Carbs (g)	Fiber (g)
2	13	2.5	na	0	200	0	2	15	3
2	12	6	0	0	380	0	4	17	3
2	12	6	0	0	360	0	4	16	3
4	2.5	0.5	0	0	370	0	8	28	5
3	13	7	0	0	340	0	4	14	2
1	10	2	0	0	280	0	2	14	3
2	10	2	0	<5	280	2	2	14	2
3	5	2.5	0	0	160	0	2	22	3
24	11	4	0	70	49	3	4	0	0
24	13	5	0	70	53	3	4	0	0
24	9	3	0	71	43	1	5	0	0
19	21	8	0	73	59	2	4	0	0
25	26	9	0	103	79	4	9	0	0
24	4	1	0	67	48	1	7	0	0
24	5	2	0	67	47	1	7	0	0
21	8	3	0	55	401	0	4	1	0
21	11	4	0	58	423	2	4	1	0
9	5	1.5	0	20	480	0	0	1	0
9	6	2	0	25	330	0	0	0	0

Pork Rinds – Potatoes (white) FOOD NAME	Portion Size	Calories	
Wise, Sweet & Mild BBQ	.625 oz	90	
POTATOES (white)			
Baked, skin & flesh	1 med	161	
Boiled, skin & flesh	2.5"	118	
Canned			
Del Monte, Au Gratin	½ c	80	
Del Monte, w/ Green Beans & Ham flavor	½ c	30	
Del Monte, New Potatoes, sliced	⅔ c	60	
S&W, New Potatoes, whole	2 pcs	60	
Frozen			
Birds Eye, Baby Whole Potatoes	7 pcs	80	
Birds Eye, Roasted Potatoes & Broccoli	⅔ c	100	
Cascadian Farm, Country Style	¾ c	50	
Cascadian Farm, Crinkle Cut French fries	18 pcs	130	
Cascadian Farm, Hash Browns	1 c	60	
Cascadian Farm, Spud Puppies	10 pcs	160	
Cascadian Farm, Wedge Cut	8 pcs	110	
McCain, Crinkle Cut	3 oz	130	
McCain, Golden Crisp	3 oz	150	
McCain, Mash bites	3 oz	170	
McCain Roasters, All-American	3 oz	120	
McCain Roasters, French Onion	3 oz	110	
McCain Roasters, Grilled Garlic & Onion	3 oz	120	
McCain Seasoned Beer Battered Wedges	3 oz	140	
McCain Seasoned Spirals	3 oz	140	

Protein (g)	Total Fat (g)	Sat. Fat (g)	Trans Fat (g)	Chol. (mg)	Sodium (mg)	Calcium (%)	Iron (%)	Carbs (g)	Fiber (g)
9	6	2	0	20	300	0	0	1	0
4	0	0	0	0	8	3	10	37	4
3	0	0	0	0	5	1	2	27	2
2	2.5	1	0	0	470	4	2	13	1
1	0	0	0	0	330	2	2	6	<1
1	0	0	0	0	360	2	2	13	2
1	0	0	0	0	360	2	2	13	2
2	0	0	0	0	25	0	2	17	1
2	4	2	0	0	470	4	10	15	1
1	0	0	0	0	10	0	2	12	1
2	4	1	0	0	15	0	4	21	2
2	0	0	0	0	10	0	4	14	1
2	7	1.5	0	0	400	0	4	23	2
2	2.5	0.5	0	0	15	0	4	21	2
2	4	0	0	0	320	0	2	21	2
2	7	0.5	0	0	400	2	4	20	2
2	7	0.5	0	0	430	0	4	24	2
2	3	0	0	0	370	0	4	21	2
2	3	0	0	0	310	0	4	20	2
2	3	0	0	0	590	0	4	22	2
2	7	1.5	2.5	0	250	0	2	17	2
2	7	0.5	0	0	390	2	4	18	2

Potatoes (white)

FOOD NAME	Portion Size	Calories
McCain Seasoned Wedges w/ Skin	3 oz	120
McCain Shoestring	45 pcs	210
McCain Steak Fries	8 pcs	120
McCain Tasti Tater Shaped	8 pcs	160
Ore-Ida, Golden Crinkles	3 oz	130
Ore-Ida, Hash Browns	¾ c	80
Ore-Ida, Shoestring	3 oz	150
Ore-Ida, Steak Fries	3 oz	110
Mixes/Boxed—Betty Crocker		
Au Gratin	½ c	100
Butter & Herb Mash	½ c	90
Cheddar & Bacon	⅔ c	100
Delux Cheesy Cheddar	⅔ c	130
Delux Creamy Scallop	½ c	140
Delux Three Cheese Mashed	½ c	150
Hash Browns	½ c	120
Homestyle Cheesy Scalloped	⅔ c	100
Homestyle Creamy Butter Mash	½ c	90
Julienne	⅓ c	90
Roasted Garlic	⅔ c	90
Specialty Scalloped	½ c	90
Specialty Sour Cream & Chives	⅔ c	100
Mixes/Boxed—Idahoan		
Mashed Four Cheese, mix	¼ c	100
Mashed Herb & Butter, mix	¼ c	110

Protein (g)	Total Fat (g)	Sat. Fat (g)	Trans Fat (g)	Chol. (mg)	Sodium (mg)	Calcium (%)	Iron (%)	Carbs (g)	Fiber (g)
2	5	0	0	0	390	0	2	17	2
2	8	0.5	0	0	340	0	4	32	3
2	3	0	0	0	330	0	2	21	2
2	7	0.5	0	0	410	0.	2	20	3
2	4	1	1.5	0	340	0	0	17	2
2	0	0	0	0	55	0	0	18	2
2	6	1	2	0	370	0	2	19	2
2	3	0.5	0.5	0	330	0	2	19	2
2	1.5	0.5	0.5	<5	610	2	2	21	1
2	1	0.5	0.5	0	400	0	2	18	1
2	1.5	0.5	0.5	<5	660	2	2	20	1
3	4.5	1.5	1	5	600	6	0	21	1
3	4.5	1.5	1	5	730	4	2	22	1
4	5	2	1.5	5	680	6	2	24	5
2	0	0	0	0	25	0	4	26	2
2	1.5	0.5	0.5	<5	570	2	2	20	2
2	1	0.5	0.5	0	370	0	2	18	1
2	1	0	0	<5	630	2	0	19	1
2	1.5	0.5	0.5	0	510	0	0	19	1
2	1	0.5	0.5	0	590	2	2	20	1
2	1	0.5	0	<5	660	2	2	20	1
2	2.5	0.5	0.5	0	550	4	2	19	1
2	2.5	0.5	0.5	0	560	2	2	20	1

Potatoes (white) – Potato Chips FOOD NAME	Portion Size	Calories
Mashed homestyle, mix	¼ c	110
Mashed, original, mix	⅓ c	80
POTATO CHIPS		
Herr's		
Bacon & Horseradish	1 oz	160
BBQ	1 oz	150
Honey Mustard	1 oz	150
Ketchup	1 oz	150
Kettle-Cooked, Jalapeno	1 oz	160
Kettle-Cooked, Original	1 oz	160
Pennsylvania Dutch Style	1 oz	150
Sour Cream & Onion	1 oz	150
Sweet Island	1 oz	150
Lay's		
Baked, Cheddar & Sour cream	1 oz	120
Baked, Original Crisps	1 oz	110
Baked, Sour Cream & Onion	1 oz	120
Deli Style, original	1 oz	150
Hot n Spicy, BBQ Flavor	1 oz	150
Kettle Cooked, Jalapeno	1 oz	140
Kettle Cooked, Mesquite BBQ	1 oz	140
Kettle Cooked, original	1 oz	150
Lightly Salted	1 oz	150
Natural Thick Cut Country BBQ	1 oz	150
Stax, Cheddar Flavored	1 oz	150

Protein (g)	Total Fat (g)	Sat. Fat (g)	Trans Fat (g)	Chol. (mg)	Sodium (mg)	Calcium (%)	Iron (%)	Carbs (g)	Fiber (g)
2	2.5	0.5	0.5	0	450	2	2	20	1
2	0	0	0	0	15	6	0	18	2
2	10	1.5	0	0	360	0	2	16	1
2	10	3	0	0	240	0	2	14	1
2	10	3	0	0	280	0	2	14	1
2	10	2.5	0	0	300	0	2	15	1
2	10	2.5	0	0	300	0	2	14	1
2	10	2.5	0	0	180	0	2	14	1
2	10	2.5	0	0	180	0	2	14	1
2	10	3	0	0	310	0	2	14	1
2	10	3	0	0	280	0	2	14	1
2	3	0.5	0	0	210	4	0	21	2
2	1.5	0	0	0	150	4	2	23	2
2	3	0	0	0	210	6	2	21	2
1	10	3	0	0	180	0	0	16	1
2	10	3	0	0	200	0	2	15	1
2	8	1	0	0	170	0	4	16	1
2	8	1	0	0	210	0	0	16	<1
2	8	1	0	0	110	0	2	18	1
2	10	1	0	0	90	0	4	15	1
2	9	1	0	0	150	0	0	15	1
1	10	2.5	0	0	190	2	2	15	1

Potato Chips – Pretzels FOOD NAME	Portion Size	Calories
Stax, Hidden Valley Ranch	1 oz	150
Stax, original	1 oz	160
Stax, Salt & Vinegar	1 oz	150
Wavy, Au Gratin	1 oz	150
Wavy, Hickory BBQ	1 oz	150
Pringles		
Chili Cheese	1 oz	160
Fat-free original	1 oz	70
Fat-free Sour Cream & Onion	1 oz	70
Loaded Baked Potato	1 oz	150
Original	1 oz	160
Ranch	1 oz	160
Sour Cream & Onion	1 oz	160
Wise		
BBQ Flavored	1 oz	150
Chipotle Flavored	1 oz	150
Kettle Cooked, Jalapeno	1 oz	140
Kettle Cooked, natural	1 oz	150
Original, Flat Cut	1 oz	150
PRETZELS		
Bachman		
Butter Twists	1 oz	110
Classic Twists	1 oz	100
Nutzels	1 oz	110
Peanut Butter Pretzels	1 oz	160

Protein (g)	Total Fat (g)	Sat. Fat (g)	Trans Fat (g)	Chol. (mg)	Sodium (mg)	Calcium (%)	Iron (%)	Carbs (g)	Fiber (g)
1	9	2.5	0	0	180	2	2	15	1
1	10	2.5	0	0	160	0	0	15	1
1	9	2.5	0	0	230	2	2	14	1
2	10	3	0	<5	200	0	0	14	1
2	9	1	0	0	210	0	0	16	1
1	11	3	0	0	230	0	2	15	1
2	0	0	0	0	160	na	na	15	2
2	0	0	0	0	190	na	na	15	2
1	10	3	0	0	170	na	na	14	<1
1	11	3	0	0	170	na	na	15	1
1	11	3	0	0	190	2	0	13	1
2	10	1.5	0	0	135	na	na	15	1
2	10	3	0	0	210	0	0	15	1
2	10	2	0	0	200	0	2	14	1
2	8	2.5	0	0	210	0	2	16	1
2	9	2.5	0	0	170	0	2	15	1
2	10	3	0	0	190	0	2	14	1
3	1	0	0	0	820	0	8	23	1
3	1	0	0	0	650	0	10	22	1
3	1	0	0	0	100	0	0	23	1
8	8	1.5	0	0	250	0	4	15	1

Pretzels

FOOD NAME	Portion Size	Calories
Sourdough Bites	1 oz	110
Wheat & Honey Pretzelmack	1 oz	110
Herr's		
Bite Size Hard	1 oz	100
Chocolate Covered Rods	7/10 oz	90
Extra Dark Specials	1 oz	110
Honey Wheat	1 oz	110
Peanut Butter Filled	10	160
Specials	1.5 oz	170
Quinlin		
Butter Flavored Braided Twists	1 oz	110
Honey Wheat Braided Twists	1 oz	110
Mini	1 oz	110
Sticks, f-f	1 oz	100
Rold Gold		
Cheddar Tiny Twists	1 oz	110
Classic Rods	1 oz	110
Classic Thins	1 oz	110
Fat-free Tiny Twists	1 oz	100
Hard Sourdough	1 oz	100
Honey Mustard Tiny Twists	1 oz	110
Land O' Lakes Butter	1 oz	110
Snyders of Hanover		
Butter Snaps	1 oz	120
Carb Fix Nibblers	1 oz	120

Protein (g)	Total Fat (g)	Sat. Fat (g)	Trans Fat (g)	Chol. (mg)	Sodium (mg)	Calcium (%)	Iron (%)	Carbs (g)	Fiber (g)
3	1	0	0	0	240	0	0	22	1
3	1	0	0	0	190	0	6	23	1
3	0	0	0	0	450	0	6	23	2
1	2.5	2	0	0	190	2	10	14	0
3	1	0	0	0	450	0	6	21	2
3	2	0	0	0	300	0	6	21	2
8	8	1.5	0	0	250	0	4	15	1
4	2	0	0	0	675	0	8	31	2
3	1	0	0	0	240	0	6	23	1
2	1	0	0	0	200	0	6	24	1
2	1	0	0	0	420	0	6	23	<1
2	0	0	0	0	490	0	6	23	<1
3	1	0	0	0	370	0	6	22	1
3	1	0	0	0	610	0	6	22	1
2	1	0	0	0	560	0	10	23	1
3	0	0	0	0	420	0	6	23	1
2	0.5	0	0	0	500	0	2	21	1
3	1	0	0	0	430	0	8	23	1
3	1.5	0	0	<5	300	0	6	22	1
3	1	0	0	0	270	0	0	25	na
5	2	0	0	0	200	0	0	21	na

FOOD NAME	Portion Size	Calories	
Homestyle	1 oz	120	
Honey Wheat Sticks	1 oz	120	
Pretzel Sesame Sticks	1 oz	120	
Sourdough Hard	1 oz	100	
12-Grain Sticks	1 oz	120	
Superpretzel—Frozen			
Pretzelfils, Mozzarella	2	130	
Pretzelfils, Pepperjack	2	130	
Pretzelfils, Pizza	2	130	
Soft pretzel, w/o added salt	1	160	
Soft Pretzel Bites, w/o added salt	5	150	
Softstix	2	130	
PRUNES/PRUNE BEVERAGE			
Knudsen, juice, organic	8 oz	170	
Old Orchard, juice cocktail	8 oz	61	
Sunsweet bite size or whole	1.5 oz	100	
Sunsweet ready to serve	⅔ c	150	
Sunsweet, juice w/ or w/o pulp	8 oz	180	
PUDDING			
Handi-Snacks, Banana or Vanilla	3.5 oz	90	
Handi-Snacks, Chocolate	3.5 oz	100	
Handi-Snacks, Chocolate, f-f	3.5 oz	90	
Handi-Snacks, Double Fudge, Rocky Road	3.5 oz	100	
Handi-Snacks, Rice	3.5 oz	140	
Jell-O			

Protein (g)	Total Fat (g)	Sat. Fat (g)	Trans Fat (g)	Chol. (mg)	Sodium (mg)	Calcium (%)	Iron (%)	Carbs (g)	Fiber (g)
3	1	0	0	0	230	0	2	25	na
3	2	0	0	0	230	0	0	24	na
3	2	0	0	0	200	0	0	23	na
3	0	0	0	0	240	0	2	22	na
3	2	0	0	0	160	0	0	23	na
6	3.5	1.5	0	5	420	8	6	20	1
5	3.5	1.5	0	5	400	6	6	21	1
5	2	1	0	5	180	6	8	22	1
5	1	0	0	0	130	0	10	34	1
3	0.5	0	0	0	115	0	8	32	1
4	3	1.5	0	10	260	4	6	22	1
1	0	0	0	0	20	4	6	20	3
0	0	0	0	0	30	10	3	16	5
1	0	0	0	0	5	2	2	24	3
2	0	0	0	0	15	2	4	37	3
2	0	0	0	0	30	2	8	43	3
1	1	0	0	0	160	2	0	20	0
1	1	1	0	0	150	2	4	23	1
2	0	0	0	0	170	na	na	21	na
1	1	1	0	0	130	2	4	23	1
3	6	1	0	0	130	2	8	19	0

Pudding FOOD NAME	Portion Size	Calories	
Banana Cream, cook & serve	½ c	80	
Banana Cream, instant	½ c	90	
Butterscotch, instant	½ c	90	
Cheesecake, instant	½ c	100	
Chocolate, cook & serve	½ c	90	
Chocolate, cook & serve, sugar free	½ c	30	
Chocolate Fudge, sugar & f-f	½ c	30	
Coconut Cream, cook & serve	½ c	90	
Lemon, instant	½ c	90	
Mixed Berry, Smoothie Snack	1 serv	100	
Oreo Cookies 'n cream	½ c	120	
Pistachio, instant	½ c	100	
Strawberry Banana, Smoothie Snack	1 serv	100	
Vanilla, cook & serve	½ c	80	
Jell-O Pudding Snacks			
Caramel, sugar free	4 oz	60	
Chocolate	4 oz	140	
Chocolate, f-f	4 oz	100	
Chocolate Vanilla Swirl	4 oz	140	
Oreo	4 oz	140	
Strawberry & Crème	4 oz	130	
Tapioca	4 oz	130	
Vanilla Caramel, f-f	4 oz	100	
Uncle Ben's			
Cinnamon & Raisin Rice Pudding	½ c	160	

Protein (g)	Total Fat (g)	Sat. Fat (g)	Trans Fat (g)	Chol. (mg)	Sodium (mg)	Calcium (%)	Iron (%)	Carbs (g)	Fiber (g)
0	0	0	0	0	180	na	na	20	0
0	0	0	0	0	360	0	0	23	0
0	0	0	0	0	390	0	0	23	0
0	0	0	0	0	360	na	na	24	0
1	0	0	0	0	110	0	4	22	1
1	0	0	0	0	110	0	6	7	1
1	0	0	0	0	300	0	4	8	1
0	2.5	2.5	0	0	150	na	na	18	1
0	0	0	0	0	310	na	na	24	0
1	2.5	1.5	0	10	40	2	0	18	0
0	1	0	0	0	390	0	2	28	0
0	0.5	0	0	0	360	0	0	23	0
1	2.5	1.5	0	10	40	2	0	18	0
0	0	0	0	0	135	na	na	20	0
1	1	1	0	0	200	10	0	13	0
2	4	1.5	0	0	190	6	4	27	1
2	0	0	0	0	180	6	2	23	1
2	4	1.5	0	0	170	6	2	26	1
2	4	1.5	0	0	170	6	2	27	1
2	3	2	0	10	85	6	0	25	0
1	3	1	0	0	150	4	0	25	0
1	0	0	0	0	230	4	0	23	0
2	1	0	0	0	180	2	6	37	0

FOOD NAME	Portion Size	Calories	
French Vanilla Rice Pudding	½ c	120	
PUMPKIN			
Fresh, cooked, no salt, mashed	1 c	49	
Libby's canned, 100% pure	½ c	40	
Libby's canned, pie mix	⅓ c	90	
Seeds, kernels, roasted, no salt	1 oz	147	
Seeds, whole, roasted, no salt	1 oz	126	
PUNCH			
Capri Sun: Fruit Punch, Grape, Orange,			
Pacific Cooler, Red Berry	200 ml	100	
Capri Sun, Splash Cooler, Strawberry,			
Tropical Punch	200 ml	90	
Hi-C: Crazy Citrus, Flashin' Fruit,			
Orange Lavaburst	200 ml	90	
Hi-C: Boppin' Strawberry, Poppin'			
Lemonade, Strawberry Kiwi, box	200 ml	100	
Hi-C Blast			
Berry Blue	8 oz	120	
Blue Watermelon, Fruit Punch, Wild			
Berry, pouch	200 ml	100	
Fruit Pow	1 bottle	180	
Orange, pouch	200 ml	90	
Raspberry Kiwi, Strawberry, pouch	200 ml	100	
Kool-Aid Bursts, Tropical Punch	200 ml	100	
Kool-Aid Mix, Tropical Punch	8 oz	60	

Protein (g)	Total Fat (g)	Sat. Fat (g)	Trans Fat (g)	Chol. (mg)	Sodium (mg)	Calcium (%)	Iron (%)	Carbs (g)	Fiber (g)
2	0	0	0	0	90	2	2	28	1
2	0	0	0	0	2	4	8	12	3
2	0.5	0	0	0	5	2	4	9	5
1	0.5	0	0	0	120	2	4	20	3
9	12	2	0	0	5	1	23	4	1
5	5	1	0	0	5	2	5	15	0
0	0	0	0	0	15	na	na	27	na
0	0	0	0	0	15	na	na	25	na
0	0	0	0	0	15	na	na	25	na
0	0	0	0	0	15	na	na	27	na
0	0	0	0	0	30	na	na	32	na
0	0	0	0	0	15	na	na	26	na
0	0	0	0	0	110	na	na	46	na
0	0	0	0	0	15	na	na	25	na
0	0	0	0	0	15	na	na	27	na
0	0	0	0	0	35	na	na	24	na
0	0	0	0	0	0	na	na	16	na

Punch – Refried Beans		
FOOD NAME	Portion Size	Calories
Minute Maid, Berry, Citrus, Grape	8 oz	120
Minute Maid, Tropical	8 oz	110
Tropicana 100% Juice Fruit Punch	10 oz	170
RADISHES, raw, slices	½ c	9
RAISINS		
Dole	¼ c	130
Sun-Maid, Baking	¼ c	110
Sun-Maid, Chocolate Covered	30 pcs	170
Sun-Maid, Chocolate Yogurt	¼ c	120
Sun-Maid, Golden or Regular	¼ c	130
Sun-Maid, Vanilla Yogurt	¼ c	130
RASPBERRIES, raw, red	1 c	64
Cascadian Farm, organic, frozen	1¼ c	70
RED BEANS		
Eden Foods, organic, canned, ½ cup	½ c	100
S&W, canned, Louisiana Style, ½ cup	½ c	80
RED SNAPPER, broiled, 3 oz	3 oz	109
REFRIED BEANS		
Eden Foods		
Black Beans, organic	½ c	110
Kidney Beans, organic	½ c	80
Pinto, organic	½ c	90
Pinto, Spicy, organic	½ c	90
Old El Paso		
Fat-free	½ c	100

Protein (g)	Total Fat (g)	Sat. Fat (g)	Trans Fat (g)	Chol. (mg)	Sodium (mg)	Calcium (%)	Iron (%)	Carbs (g)	Fiber (g)
0	0	0	0	0	15	na	na	32	na
0	0	0	0	0	15	na	na	30	na
0	0	0	0	0	30	na	na	40	na
0	0	0	0	0	23	1	1	2	1
1	0	0	0	0	10	2	6	31	2
1	0	0	0	0	5	2	4	27	2
2	6	4	0	5	20	4	4	25	1
1	4	3.5	0	0	20	4	2	22	1
1	0	0	0	0	10	2	6	31	2
1	5	4	0	0	20	4	2	21	1
1	1	0	0	0	1	3	5	15	8
1	1	0	0	0	0	2	4	16	7
6	0.5	0	0	0	25	4	8	17	5
6	0	0	0	0	480	4	10	20	5
22	1	0	0	0	40	3	1	48	0
6	1.5	0	0	0	180	4	15	18	7
7	1	0	0	0	180	4	10	15	6
6	1	0	0	0	180	4	8	19	7
6	1	0	0	0	180	4	8	19	7
6	0	0	0	0	580	4	10	18	6

Refried Beans – Rice FOOD NAME	Portion Size	Calories	
Fat-free, Spicy	½ c	100	
Traditional	½ c	100	
Vegetarian	½ c	100	
w/ Sausage	½ c	200	
Taco-Bell			
Original, f-f	½ c	110	
Vegetarian	½ c	140	
RELISH			
Claussen, Sweet	1 Tbs	15	
Vlasic, Dill	1 Tbs	5	
Vlasic, Relish Mixers	1 Tbs	10	
Vlasic, Specialty Blend	1 Tbs	20	
Vlasic, Sweet	1 Tbs	15	
RHUBARB, raw, diced	⅔ c	26	
Frozen (Dole)	1 c	30	
RICE			
Long Grain, prep	1 c	194	
Medium or Short Grain, prep	1 c	242	
Carolina, Extra Long Grain White, prep	¾ c	150	
Carolina, Gold (parboiled), prep	1 c	160	
Carolina, Jasmine, prep	¾ c	160	
Carolina, Long Grain Brown, prep	¾ c	150	
Minute Rice, Instant Long Grain Brown, prep	¾ c	170	

Protein (g)	Total Fat (g)	Sat. Fat (g)	Trans Fat (g)	Chol. (mg)	Sodium (mg)	Calcium (%)	Iron (%)	Carbs (g)	Fiber (g)
6	0	0	0	0	570	4	10	18	6
6	0.5	0	0	0	570	4	10	18	6
6	1	0	0	0	560	4	10	17	6
7	13	5	0	10	360	4	10	14	4
7	0	0	0	0	460	na	na	21	6
5	3	0.5	0	0	530	na	na	23	7
0	0	0	0	0	85	na	na	3	na
0	0	0	0	0	240	na	na	1	na
0	0	0	0	0	55	na	na	5	na
0	0	0	0	0	220	na	na	5	na
0	0	0	0	0	140	na	na	4	na
1	0	0	0	0	0	8	0	4	2
0	0	0	0	0	0	25	2	7	3
5	1	0	0	0	3	3	16	41	1
4	0	0	0	0	0	1	15	53	1
3	0	0	0	0	0	0	8	35	0
3	0	0	0	0	0	0	8	37	<1
3	0	0	0	0	0	0	8	36	0
3	1	0	0	0	0	0	8	32	1
4	1.5	0	0	0	10	0	2	34	2

FOOD NAME	Portion Size	Calories	
Minute Rice, Instant Long Grain			
White, prep	¾ c	160	
Uncle Ben's Fast & Natural Brown, prep	1 c	190	
Uncle Ben's Instant White, prep	1 c	190	
Uncle Ben's Long Grain & Wild, prep	1 c	240	
RICE MIXES			
Betty Crocker Bowl Appetit			
Cheddar Broccoli Rice	1 bowl	290	
Herb Chicken Vegetable	1 bowl	260	
Teriyaki Rice	1 bowl	260	
Carolina			
Authentic Spanish, mix	⅓ c	180	
Black Bean & Rice, mix	⅓ c	200	
Chicken & Rice, mix	⅓ c	190	
Classic Pilaf, mix	⅓ c	190	
Saffron Yellow, mix	⅓ c	190	
Spicy Yellow, mix	⅓ c	180	
Knorr-Lipton			
Beef, mix	½ c	230	
Cajun Style, Dirty Rice, mix	½ c	250	
Cajun Style, Garlic Butter, mix	½ c	260	
Cajun Style, New Orleans, mix	½ c	250	
Cajun Style, Red Rice & Beans, mix	½ c	290	
Cheddar Broccoli, mix	½ c	230	
Chicken Broccoli, mix	½ c	220	

Protein (g)	Total Fat (g)	Sat. Fat (g)	Trans Fat (g)	Chol. (mg)	Sodium (mg)	Calcium (%)	Iron (%)	Carbs (g)	Fiber (g)
3	0	0	0	0	5	0	10	36	1
4	1.5	0	0	0	20	0	2	42	2
3	0.5	0	0	0	15	2	10	43	1
5	3.5	0	0	0	500	4	8	44	1
8	7	2.5	2	10	950	15	8	51	2
7	5	1.5	1	15	780	2	10	49	2
7	3	0.5	1	0	1160	2	10	54	2
4	0	0	0	0	650	0	10	42	1
7	1.5	0	0	0	930	8	15	39	5
3	0	0	0	0	970	10	10	42	<1
5	0	0	0	0	810	0	8	43	1
4	0	0	0	0	970	4	10	43	<1
4	0.5	0	0	0	1150	2	10	41	<1
6	0.5	0	0	0	960	2	15	49	1
8	1.5	0	0	5	820	4	15	50	2
7	4	2	0	10	780	2	15	48	1
7	1.5	0	0	0	720	4	15	50	2
9	1	0	0	0	540	0	15	61	5
6	1.5	0.5	0	<5	860	6	15	47	2
6	1	0	0	<5	800	2	15	45	2

Rice Mixes

FOOD NAME	Portion Size	Calories
Herb & Butter, mix	½ c	250
Rice Medley, mix	½ c	210
Rice Pilaf, mix	½ c	220
Near East		
Brown Rice Pilaf, mix	¼ c	180
Long Grain & Wild, mix	⅓ c	190
Rice Pilaf Toasted Almond, mix	¼ c	200
Sundried Tomato & Basil, mix	⅓ c	240
Rice-a-Roni		
Beef, mix	⅓ c	230
Broccoli Au Gratin, mix	⅓ c	260
Cheesy Italian Herb, mix	⅓ c	260
Chicken, mix	⅓ c	230
Chicken & Garlic, mix	⅓ c	190
Fried, mix	⅓ c	240
Herb & Butter, mix	⅓ c	240
Pilaf, mix	⅓ c	230
Spanish, mix	⅓ c	180
Uncle Ben's		
Brown & Wild, Mushroom recipe	1 c	200
Brown & Wild, Roasted Garlic	1 c	200
Brown & Wild, Vegetables & Herbs	1 c	200
Country Inn, Broccoli Au Gratin	1 c	200
Country Inn, Chicken & Vegetables	1 c	200
Country Inn, Oriental Fried	1 c	200

Protein (g)	Total Fat (g)	Sat. Fat (g)	Trans Fat (g)	Chol. (mg)	Sodium (mg)	Calcium (%)	Iron (%)	Carbs (g)	Fiber (g)
6	4.5	2.5	0	10	850	2	15	46	1
6	1	0	0	<5	780	2	15	43	1
6	2	1	0	<5	870	0	10	43	1
5	1	0	0	0	660	2	4	41	3
5	0.5	0	0	0	800	2	4	43	2
5	3	0	0	0	640	2	4	40	2
6	0.5	0	0	0	1030	2	6	54	2
7	1	0	0	0	1020	10	10	50	2
7	6	3	0	5	870	10	15	46	2
7	6	2	na	5	830	20	10	46	2
7	1	0	0	0	1070	10	15	51	2
5	0.5	0	0	0	740	10	15	41	2
7	1.5	0	0	0	1390	10	10	49	2
5	1.5	0.5	0	0	1070	10	10	52	1
7	1	0	0	0	1110	10	10	51	2
5	0.5	0	0	0	980	10	15	40	2
6	1.5	0	0	0	590	2	6	41	3
5	1	0	0	0	750	4	15	42	1
5	1.5	0	0	0	800	6	15	42	1
4	2	1	0	0	790	4	10	43	1
5	1.5	0.5	0	0	720	2	20	41	1
6	1	0	0	0	580	2	20	42	1

Rice Mixes – Rice Cakes/Crackers/Chips FOOD NAME	Portion Size	Calories	
Country Inn, Three Cheese	1 c	200	
Flavorful, Garlic & Butter	1 c	200	
Flavorful, Parmesan & Butter	1 c	200	
Flavorful, Tomato & Herb	1 c	200	
Ready Rice, Roasted Chicken	1 c	230	
Ready Rice, Spanish	1 c	240	
Ready Rice, Teriyaki	1 c	260	
RICE BEVERAGES			
Rice Dream, Carob	8 oz	150	
Rice Dream, Chocolate Enriched	8 oz	170	
Rice Dream, original	8 oz	120	
Rice Dream, Vanilla	8 oz	130	
Rice Dream, Vanilla Heartwise	8 oz	140	
Westbrae, plain	8 oz	100	
Westbrae, Vanilla	8 oz	120	
RICE CAKES/CRACKERS/CHIPS			
Eden Foods			
Brown Rice Chips	25 pcs	150	
Brown Rice Crackers	8 pcs	120	
Nori Maki Rice Crackers	15 pcs	110	
Quaker Rice Cakes			
Apple Cinnamon	1	50	
Butter Popped Corn	1	35	
Chocolate Crunch	1	60	
Peanut Butter Chocolate Chip	1	60	

Protein (g)	Total Fat (g)	Sat. Fat (g)	Trans Fat (g)	Chol. (mg)	Sodium (mg)	Calcium (%)	Iron (%)	Carbs (g)	Fiber (g)
6	2	1	0	5	800	6	15	40	1
5	0.5	0	0	0	750	4	2	44	<1
5	1	0	0	0	550	6	10	43	1
4	0.5	0	0	0	850	4	2	45	<1
5	4	0	0	0	960	4	6	44	1
5	3.5	0	0	0	500	4	0	44	1
7	3	0.5	1	0	1160	2	10	54	2
1	2.5	0	0	0	100	2	4	32	0
1	3	0	0	0	115	30	6	36	0
1	2	0	0	0	90	2	0	25	0
1	2	0	0	0	90	30	0	28	0
1	2	0	0	0	80	30	2	30	3
1	2.5	0	0	0	60	25	2	18	0
1	2.5	0	0	0	65	25	2	22	0
2	7	1.5	0	0	100	0	0	19	0
3	2	0	0	0	230	2	4	22	2
3	0	0	0	0	160	4	2	24	2
0	0	0	0	0	0	0	0	11	0
1	0	0	0	0	45	0	0	8	0
1	1	0	0	0	35	0	0	12	0
1	1	0	0	0	70	0	0	12	0

Rice Cakes/Crackers/Chips – Rolls (nonsweet) FOOD NAME	Portion Size	Calories	
White Cheddar	1	45	
RICE PUDDING; see "Pudding"			
ROCKFISH, Pacific, baked	3 oz	103	
ROLLS (nonsweet)			
Pepperidge Farm			
Carb Style, Hamburger	1	110	
Farmhouse Country Wheat	1	220	
Frankfurter	1	140	
Hamburger	1	120	
Hot & Crusty French	1	100	
Hot & Crusty 7 Grain	1	110	
Onion Sandwich Bun	1	150	
Parker House Dinner	1	80	
Soft 100% Whole Wheat Kaiser	1	200	
Soft Country Style Dinner	1	90	
Soft Hoagie	1	210	
Soft White Kaiser	1	210	
Pillsbury			
Crescent Big & Buttery	1	170	
Crescent Big & Flaky	1	180	
Crescent Butterflake	1	110	
Crescent Original	1	110	
Dinner, White Quick	1	110	
Freezer to Microwave, White Dinner	1	150	
Freezer to Oven Crusty French	1	100	

Protein (g)	Total Fat (g)	Sat. Fat (g)	Trans Fat (g)	Chol. (mg)	Sodium (mg)	Calcium (%)	Iron (%)	Carbs (g)	Fiber (g)
1	0.5	0	0	0	160	0	0	8	0
20	2	0	0	37	65	1	3	0	0
7	1	0	0	<5	190	4	6	17	3
8	4.5	1	na	0	310	8	10	36	1
5	2.5	1	na	0	270	6	6	24	<1
5	2	0.5	na	0	180	2	6	22	1
3	1	0	0	0	180	2	4	19	0
4	2	0.5	na	0	200	4	8	21	2
6	2.5	0.5	na	0	95	2	2	14	<1
3	2	0.5	na	0	95	2	2	14	<1
9	2.5	1	na	0	370	6	10	35	3
3	1.5	0	na	0	150	2	6	17	1
7	6	1.5	na	0	350	6	8	35	2
9	2.5	0.5	na	0	340	6	10	37	<1
3	10	2.5	2.5	0	370	0	6	20	<1
3	10	2.5	2.5	0	370	0	6	20	<1
2	6	2	1.5	0	220	0	4	11	0
2	6	2	1.5	0	220	0	4	11	0
5	2	0.5	0.5	0	270	0	6	18	<1
4	4	1	1	0	220	0	6	26	<1
4	1.5	0	0	0	200	0	6	18	<1

Rolls (nonsweet) – Salad Dressing FOOD NAME	Portion Size	Calories	
Freezer to Oven, Dinner, Garlic	1	140	
Freezer to Oven, Dinner, Whole Wheat	1	90	
Sara Lee			
Classic Heart Healthy Wheat Hamburger	1	190	
Classic Wheat Buns	1	200	
Classic White Buns	1	200	
Gourmet Hot Dog	1	120	
ROLLS (Sweet)—Pillsbury			
Freezer to Oven Sweet, Cinnamon	1	290	
Grands! Extra Rich Cinnamon w/ Icing	1	320	
Grands! Sweet Cinnamon w/ Icing	1	310	
Grands! Sweet Cinnamon w/ Icing, reduced fat	1	300	
Grands! Sweet Orange	1	330	
Sweet Rolls, Caramel	1	170	
Sweet Rolls, Cinnamon w/ Cream Cheese Icing	1	150	
Sweet Rolls, Cinnamon Raisin w/ Icing	1	170	
Sweet Rolls, Cinnamon w/ Icing	1	150	
Sweet Rolls, Cinnamon w/ Icing, sugar free	1	110	
Sweet Rolls, Golden Homestyle Cinnamon	1	130	
Sweet Rolls, Orange w/ Icing	1	170	
SALAD DRESSING			
Annie's Naturals			
Artichoke Parmesan	2 Tbs	130	

Protein (g)	Total Fat (g)	Sat. Fat (g)	Trans Fat (g)	Chol. (mg)	Sodium (mg)	Calcium (%)	Iron (%)	Carbs (g)	Fiber (g)
3	6	1.5	1	0	220	0	6	17	<1
4	1	0	0	0	170	0	4	17	3
7	2.5	0.5	0	0	370	6	10	37	3
7	3.5	1	0	0	390	6	15	38	3
6	3	1	0	0	390	10	10	37	1
4	1.5	0	0	0	230	4	6	23	<1
6	10	2.5	2.5	15	720	2	10	46	1
5	10	2.5	3	0	690	2	10	54	1
5	9	2	2.5	0	640	2	10	54	1
5	6	1.5	1.5	0	650	2	10	56	1
5	11	2.5	3	0	650	2	10	53	1
2	7	1.5	2.5	0	320	0	6	24	<1
2	5	1.5	2	0	340	0	4	23	<1
2	6	1.5	2	0	320	0	6	26	<1
2	5	1.5	2	0	340	0	4	23	<1
2	3.5	1	1	0	360	0	4	23	3
2	3	1	1	0	360	0	6	24	<1
2	7	1.5	2	0	340	0	6	25	<1
1	13	1.5	0	<5	250	2	0	1	0

Salad Dressing FOOD NAME	Portion Size	Calories	
Balsamic Vinaigrette	2 Tbs	100	
Thousand Island	2 Tbs	90	
Woodstock	2 Tbs	110	
Kraft			
Catalina, f-f	2 Tbs	35	
Creamy French	2 Tbs	160	
Creamy Italian	2 Tbs	110	
Italian, f-f	2 Tbs	15	
Ranch	2 Tbs	170	
Ranch Garlic	2 Tbs	180	
Roka Blue Cheese	2 Tbs	150	
Thousand Island	2 Tbs	120	
Three Cheese Italian	2 Tbs	130	
Zesty Italian	2 Tbs	110	
Kraft—Carb Well			
Classic Caesar	2 Tbs	110	
Creamy French	2 Tbs	100	
Italian	2 Tbs	70	
Light Buttermilk Ranch	2 Tbs	60	
Light Italian	2 Tbs	20	
Ranch	2 Tbs	110	
Roka Blue Cheese	2 Tbs	120	
Kraft—Light Done Right			
Creamy French	2 Tbs	80	
Italian	2 Tbs	40	

Protein (g)	Total Fat (g)	Sat. Fat (g)	Trans Fat (g)	Chol. (mg)	Sodium (mg)	Calcium (%)	Iron (%)	Carbs (g)	Fiber (g)
0	10	0.5	0	0	75	0	0	3	0
<1	7	1	0	0	140	0	0	5	0
0	11	1	0	0	260	0	2	1	0
0	0	0	0	0	320	0	0	8	1
0	15	2.5	0	0	270	0	0	5	0
0	11	1.5	0	0	250	0	0	2	0
0	0	0	0	0	430	0	0	4	0
0	18	3	0	10	280	0	0	2	0
0	19	3	0	10	270	0	0	1	0
1	13	2.5	0	5	310	0	0	2	1
0	10	1.5	0	10	310	0	0	5	0
1	11	2.5	0	0	010	0	0	0	0
0	11	1.5	0	0	530	0	0	2	0
1	11	2	0	5	310	0	0	0	0
1	11	1.5	0	5	360	0	0	0	0
0	8	1	0	0	300	0	0	0	0
1	6	1	0	5	430	0	0	0	0
0	1.5	0	0	0	490	0	0	0	0
0	11	1.5	0	5	310	0	0	0	0
0	13	2	0	5	260	0	0	0	0
0	4.5	0.5	0	0	280	0	0	9	0
0	3	0.5	0	0	270	0	0	3	0

Salad Dressing FOOD NAME	Portion Size	Calories	
Ranch	2 Tbs	80	
Roka Blue	2 Tbs	70	
Zesty Italian, reduced fat	2 Tbs	25	
Kraft—Special Collection			
Caesar Italian w/ Oregano	2 Tbs	100	
Creamy Poppyseed	2 Tbs	130	
Greek Vinaigrette	2 Tbs	110	
Italian Pesto	2 Tbs	70	
Italian Vinaigrette	2 Tbs	50	
Sun Dried Tomato	2 Tbs	60	
Tangy Tomato Bacon	2 Tbs	130	
Newman's Own			
Caesar	2 Tbs	150	
Olive Oil & Vinegar	2 Tbs	150	
Ranch	2 Tbs	140	
2000 Island	2 Tbs	140	
Three Cheese Balsamic	1 Tbs	100	
Seven Seas			
Creamy Italian	2 Tbs	110	
Green Goddess	2 Tbs	130	
Red Wine Vinaigrette	2 Tbs	90	
Viva Italian	2 Tbs	90	
Viva Italian, reduced fat	2 Tbs	45	
South Beach Diet			
Italian w/ Extra Olive Oil	2 Tbs	60	

Protein (g)	Total Fat (g)	Sat. Fat (g)	Trans Fat (g)	Chol. (mg)	Sodium (mg)	Calcium (%)	Iron (%)	Carbs (g)	Fiber (g)
0	7	0.5	0	10	300	0	0	3	0
1	6	1	0	5	290	0	0	3	0
0	1.5	0	0	0	470	0	0	2	0
1	10	1.5	0	0	470	2	0	2	0
0	10	2	0	0	250	0	0	8	0
0	11	1.5	0	0	320	0	0	25	0
1	5	0.5	0	0	270	2	0	5	0
0	4	0	0	0	420	0	0	4	0
0	5	0.5	0	0	340	0	0	4	0
1	10	1.5	0	0	410	0	0	8	0
1	18	1.5	0	0	420	2	0	1	0
1	16	2.5	0	0	150	na	na	1	0
0	15	2	0	10	250	na	na	2	0
0	14	2	0	10	260	na	na	4	0
0	11	1.5	0	0	380	2	0	2	0
0	12	2	0	0	510	na	na	2	0
0	13	2	0	0	260	na	na	1	0
0	9	0.5	0	0	480	na	na	2	0
0	9	1	0	0	380	na	na	2	0
0	4	0.5	0	0	370	na	na	2	0
0	4.5	0	0	0	300	0	0	3	0

Salad Dressing FOOD NAME	Portion Size	Calories	
Ranch	2 Tbs	70	
Wishbone			
Chunky Blue Cheese	2 Tbs	150	
Creamy Caesar	2 Tbs	170	
Deluxe French	2 Tbs	120	
Garlic Ranch	2 Tbs	140	
Russian	2 Tbs	120	
Sweet 'n spicy	2 Tbs	130	
Thousand Island	2 Tbs	130	
Wishbone—Fat Free			
Chunky Blue Cheese	2 Tbs	35	
Italian	2 Tbs	20	
Ranch	2 Tbs	30	
Wishbone—Just2Good			
Blue Cheese	2 Tbs	50	
Creamy Caesar	2 Tbs	50	
Deluxe French	2 Tbs	50	
Honey Dijon	2 Tbs	50	
Ranch	2 Tbs	40	
Thousand Island	2 Tbs	50	
Wishbone—Salad Spritzers			
Balsamic Breeze	10 sprays	10	
Italian Vinaigrette	10 sprays	10	
Red Wine Mist	10 sprays	10	
Wishbone—Western			

Protein (g)	Total Fat (g)	Sat. Fat (g)	Trans Fat (g)	Chol. (mg)	Sodium (mg)	Calcium (%)	Iron (%)	Carbs (g)	Fiber (g)
1	7	1	0	0	300	na	na	2	0
0	15	2.5	0	5	260	0	0	2	0
<1	18	3	0	10	300	0	2	1	0
0	11	1.5	0	0	170	0	0	5	0
0	15	2	0	0	310	0	0	2	0
0	6	1	0	0	360	0	0	14	0
0	12	2	0	0	330	0	0	6	0
0	12	2	0	10	330	0	4	5	0
<1	0	0	0	0	280	0	0	7	<1
0	0	0	0	0	350	0	0	4	0
0	0	0	0	0	280	0	0	7	<1
<1	2	0.5	0	0	310	0	0	6	0
2	0.5	0	0	10	310	0	0	7	0
0	2	0	0	0	250	0	0	8	<1
0	2	0	0	0	250	0	0	8	<1
0	2	0	0	0	290	0	0	5	0
0	2	0	0	5	290	0	0	9	0
0	1	0	0	0	95	0	0	1	0
0	1	0	0	0	100	0	0	1	0
0	1	0	0	0	95	0	0	1	0

Salad Dressing – Salsa FOOD NAME	Portion Size	Calories	
With Bacon Flavor	2 Tbs	140	
With Blue Cheese	2 Tbs	140	
Fat-free	2 Tbs	50	
Original	2 Tbs	160	
SALAMI			
Hebrew National, beef	3 pcs	150	
Oscar Mayer, cotto	1 oz	70	
Oscar Mayer, cotto beef	1 oz	60	
Oscar Mayer, hard	1 oz	100	
SALMON			
Canned, blueback (Bumblebee)	2.2 oz	110	
Canned, keta (Bumblebee)	2.2 oz	90	
Canned, pink (Bumblebee)	2.2 oz	90	
Canned, red (Bumblebee)	2.2 oz	110	
Canned, pink (Chicken of the Sea)	2 oz	60	
Canned, traditional red (Chicken of the Sea)	¼ c	110	
Fresh, Atlantic Wild, cooked dry	3 oz	155	
Fresh, Chinook Wild, cooked dry	3 oz	196	
Smoked Pacific (Chicken of the Sea)	1 pkg	120	
Steak w/Orange Glaze (Chicken of the Sea)	1pkg	170	
SALSA			
Muir Glen organic, Black Bean & Corn	2 Tbs	20	
Muir Glen organic, Mild	2 Tbs	10	

Protein (g)	Total Fat (g)	Sat. Fat (g)	Trans Fat (g)	Chol. (mg)	Sodium (mg)	Calcium (%)	Iron (%)	Carbs (g)	Fiber (g)
0	11	1.5	0	0	240	0	0	10	0
<1	12	2	0	0	240	0	0	9	0
0	0	0	0	0	280	0	0	12	0
0	12	1.5	0	0	230	0	0	11	0
8	13	6	0	35	420	0	0	0	0
4	6	2	0	25	280	0	4	1	0
4	4.5	2	0	20	360	0	4	1	0
7	8	3	0	25	51	0	2	1	0
13	7	1.5	0	40	270	10	2	0	0
13	4	1	0	40	270	10	2	0	0
12	5	1	0	40	270	10	2	0	0
13	7	1.5	0	40	70	10	2	0	0
10	2	1	0	20	280	0	2	0	0
13	7	2	0	40	270	10	2	0	0
22	7	1	0	60	58	1	5	0	0
22	11	3	0	72	51	2	4	0	0
21	3.5	1	0	45	490	2	4	1	0
25	1.5	0.5	0	40	470	2	2	14	0
<1	0	0	0	0	135	0	2	4	0
0	0	0	0	0	130	0	0	3	0

Salsa – Sauces FOOD NAME	Portion Size	Calories	
Newman's Own, Black Bean & Corn	2 Tbs	20	
Newman's Own, Mango	2 Tbs	20	
Newman's Own, Natural Bandito Mild	2 Tbs	10	
Newman's Own, Peach	2 Tbs	25	
Newman's Own, Tequila Lime	2 Tbs	15	
Old El Paso, Cheese 'n Salsa Medium	2 Tbs	40	
Old El Paso, Thick 'n Chunky, Mild	2 Tbs	10	
Pace, Chunky	2 Tbs	10	
Pace, Lime & Garlic Chunky	2 Tbs	15	
Taco Bell, Salso Con Queso	2 Tbs	40	
Taco Bell, Thick 'n Chunky, Mild	2 Tbs	15	
SARDINES			
Bumblebee, in mustard	3.75 oz	130	
Bumblebee, in soya oil	3.75 oz	130	
Bumblebee, in water	3.75 oz	120	
Chicken of the Sea, smoked, in oil	1 can	190	
Chicken of the Sea, in tomato	1 can	130	
Chicken of the Sea, in water	1 can	100	
Crown Prince, brisling in mustard	1 can	210	
Crown Prince, brisling in soy oil	1 can	200	
Crown Prince, brisling in tomato	1 can	210	
SAUCES			
A1 Sauce			
Jamaican Jerk Steak Sauce	2 Tbs	25	
New York Steak Sauce	2 Tbs	20	

Protein (g)	Total Fat (g)	Sat. Fat (g)	Trans Fat (g)	Chol. (mg)	Sodium (mg)	Calcium (%)	Iron (%)	Carbs (g)	Fiber (g)
1	0	0	0	0	140	2	2	5	2
1	0	0	0	0	140	2	2	5	2
0	0	0	0	0	105	na	na	2	1
0	0	0	0	0	90	0	0	6	<1
0	0	0	0	0	170	2	2	3	0
<1	3	1	1	0	200	2	0	3	0
0	0	0	0	0	230	0	0	3	0
0	0	0	0	0	230	0	0	2	<1
0	0	0	0	0	210	0	0	3	<1
1	3	0.5	0	5	260	2	0	3	0
1	0	0	0	0	210	0	0	3	0
15	6	1.5	0	40	490	15	6	0	1
13	9	2	0	35	340	10	2	0	0
13	7	2	0	35	340	10	2	0	0
12	14	6	0	45	430	20	4	2	0
17	6	2	0	60	490	30	6	2	2
13	4	2	0	45	430	20	4	2	0
14	16	6	0	45	710	20	8	<1	<1
16	16	4.5	0	65	390	20	6	0	<1
16	16	6	0	50	600	20	6	0	<1
0	0.5	0	0	0	190	na	na	5	0
0	0	0	0	0	230	na	na	5	0

Sauces – Sausage / FOOD NAME	Portion Size	Calories	
Teriyaki Steak Sauce	2 Tbs	20	
Eden Foods			
Shoyu Soy Sauce	1 Tbs	15	
Tamari Soy Sauce	1 Tbs	10	
Kraft			
Cocktail	2 Tbs	60	
Coleslaw Maker	2 Tbs	110	
Sweet & Sour	2 Tbs	60	
Tarter Sauce	2 Tbs	70	
Old El Paso			
Enchilada, mild	¼ c	25	
Taco Sauce, mild	1 Tbs	5	
Zesty Ranch Sauce	2 Tbs	70	
SAUERKRAUT			
Del Monte	2 Tbs	0	
Del Monte, Bavarian	2 Tbs	15	
Eden, organic	½ c	25	
S&W	2 Tbs	0	
SAUSAGE			
Armour			
Brown & Serve, Bacon Flavor	3 links	180	
Brown & Serve, Beef	3 links	230	
Brown & Serve, Country Recipe	3 links	210	
Brown & Serve, Lite Original	3 links	120	
Brown & Serve, Turkey	3 links	120	

Protein (g)	Total Fat (g)	Sat. Fat (g)	Trans Fat (g)	Chol. (mg)	Sodium (mg)	Calcium (%)	Iron (%)	Carbs (g)	Fiber (g)
0	0	0	0	0	30	na	na	5	0
2	0	0	0	0	1010	0	0	2	0
2	0	0	0	0	990	0	4	2	0
1	0.5	0	0	0	900	0	4	11	1
0	9	1.5	0	10	230	0	0	7	0
0	0	0	0	0	125	0	0	13	0
0	6	1	0	5	230	0	0	4	0
0	1	0	0	0	270	0	0	3	0
0	0	0	0	0	90	0	0	1	0
0	6	1	1	<5	330	0	0	2	0
0	0	0	0	0	180	0	0	0	<1
0	0	0	0	0	180	0	0	4	0
2	0	0	0	0	580	4	6	4	3
0	0	0	0	0	180	0	0	1	0
9	16	6	na	45	630	4	2	2	0
6	22	10	na	40	460	0	4	1	0
7	19	7	na	45	500	4	2	2	0
3	8	3	na	45	410	4	2	3	0
10	8	2.5	na	35	370	4	4	2	0

FOOD NAME	Portion Size	Calories	
Chicken Vienna Sausage	3 links	90	
Bob Evans			
Pork Sausage Links, Maple	2 links	130	
Pork Sausage Links, Original	2 links	130	
Hillshire			
Smoked, Beef	2 oz	190	
Smoked, Brat	1 link	240	
Jimmy Dean			
Pork Sausage Link, original	3 links	260	
Pork Sausage, Maple Patties	2 pcs	260	
Libby's, Vienna	3 links	130	
Lightlife (soy)			
Gimme Lean Sausage Style	2 oz	50	
Smart Brats	1 link	120	
Smart Links Country Breakfast	2 links	100	
Louis Rich, Turkey Sausage	3 oz	120	
Oscar Mayer			
Pork Sausage Links	2 links		
Pork Sausage Patties			
SCALLIONS, fresh, chopped	1 c	32	
SCALLOPS, bay or sea	1 oz	32	
Mrs. Paul's Fried Breaded Scallops	13 pcs	260	
SESAME			
Arrowhead Mills, Tahini (Sesame Spread)	2 Tbs	190	
Maranatha Tahini Butter, no salt	2 Tbs	190	

Protein (g)	Total Fat (g)	Sat. Fat (g)	Trans Fat (g)	Chol. (mg)	Sodium (mg)	Calcium (%)	Iron (%)	Carbs (g)	Fiber (g)
5	7	2	0	40	480	6	4	1	0
7	11	4	0	25	270	0	4	2	0
8	10	4	0	25	290	0	4	0	0
7	17	8	1	40	460	0	4	1	0
10	21	8	0	50	660	0	6	3	0
10	24	8	0	50	290	0	2	2	0
8	23	8	0	50	440	2	2	6	0
5	12	5	0	40	260	4	0	1	4
8	0	0	0	0	330	na	na	4	2
13	5	0	0	0	580	na	na	5	1
10	3.5	0.5	0	0	580	na	na	8	4
12	8	2.5	0	55	430	na	na	1	0
2	0	0	0	0	16	7	8	7	3
7	0	0	0	15	75	3	5	15	0
12	11	4	0	25	700	4	4	28	0
8	18	2.5	0	0	10	4	15	3	<1
6	16	2	0	0	5	2	10	9	2

FOOD NAME	Portion Size	Calories	
SHAD, American, cooked dry	3 oz	214	
SHERBET			
Breyers, Orange	½ c	130	
Breyers, Rainbow	½ c	130	
Dreyer's, Berry Rainbow or Tropical Rainbow	½ c	130	
Dreyer's, Key Lime	½ c	130	
Dreyer's, Orange Cream	½ c	120	
Dreyer's, Raspberry or Strawberry	½ c	130	
Dreyers, Swiss Orange	½ c	150	
SHRIMP			
Canned, regular (Bumblebee)	¼ c	40	
Frozen, premium, cooked (Chicken of the Sea)	3 oz	80	
Frozen, premium, raw (Chicken of the Sea)	4 oz	120	
SNACK MIX			
Chex, Bold Party Blend	½ c	140	
Chex Mix, Cheddar	⅔ c	130	
Chex Mix, Honey Nut	½ c	130	
Chex Mix, Hot 'n Spicy	⅔ c	130	
Chex Mix, Peanut Lovers	½ c	140	
Chex Mix, Summer Ranch	⅔ c	120	
Chex Mix, Traditional	⅔ c	130	
Chex Trail	½ c	140	
Chocolate Peanut Butter	⅔ c	150	

Protein (g)	Total Fat (g)	Sat. Fat (g)	Trans Fat (g)	Chol. (mg)	Sodium (mg)	Calcium (%)	Iron (%)	Carbs (g)	Fiber (g)
18	15	0	0	82	55	5	6	0	0
1	1.5	1	0	5	25	4	0	28	0
1	1.5	1	0	5	25	4	0	27	0
1	1.5	0.5	0	5	35	4	0	29	0
1	1.5	0.5	0	0	05	4	0	20	0
2	2	1	0	10	40	4	0	23	0
1	1	0.5	0	4	35	4	0	28	0
1	3	2.5	0	5	40	4	0	30	0
10	0	0	0	0	430	6	2	0	0
18	1	0	0	.165	190	2	15	0	0
23	2	0	0	170	170	6	10	1	0
3	6	1	0.5	0	390	0	2	20	<1
2	4	1	0	0	370	2	2	22	<1
2	4	0.5	0	0	250	0	6	23	1
2	4	1	0.5	0	420	0	2	22	1
3	6	1	0	0	340	0	4	19	1
3	3	0.5	0	0	430	0	2	21	<1
2	4	0.5	0	0	380	0	2	22	1
2	4.5	1.5	0	0	230	0	2	22	1
3	5	1.5	0	0	270	0	2	23	<1

Snack Mix – Soft Drinks FOOD NAME	Portion Size	Calories	
Chocolate Turtle	⅔ c	150	
Eden Foods, All Mixed Up	3 Tbs	160	
Gardetto's Italian Cheese Blend	½ c	140	
Gardetto's Mustard Pretzel Mix	½ c	130	
Gardetto's Snack Mix, original	½ c	150	
Gardetto's Snack Mix, original, reduced fat	½ c	130	
Nabisco, Cheddar	1 oz		
Nabisco, traditional			
Planters, Trail Mix, Fruit & Nut	1 oz	140	
Planters Trail Mix, Golden Nut Crunch	1 oz	160	
Planters Trail Mix, Mixed Nuts & Raisins	1 oz	150	
Planters Trail Mix, Nut & Chocolate	1 oz	160	
Planters Trail Mix, Spicy Nuts	1 oz	150	
SOFT DRINKS			
Canada Dry			
Club Soda	8 oz	0	
Ginger Ale	8 oz	80	
Tonic Water	8 oz	90	
Dr Pepper, original	12 oz	160	
Hansen's Natural Sodas			
Black Cherry, Grapefruit, Orange			
Mango, Raspberry, Vanilla Cola	12 oz	160	
Key Lime, Mandarin Lime	12 oz	130	
IBC			
Black Cherry	12 oz	180	

Protein (g)	Total Fat (g)	Sat. Fat (g)	Trans Fat (g)	Chol. (mg)	Sodium (mg)	Calcium (%)	Iron (%)	Carbs (g)	Fiber (g)
2	5	2	0	<5	280	0	2	23	<1
8	12	2	0	0	70	0	8	7	4
3	4	1	1	0	320	0	0	20	<1
3	2	0	0	0	220	0	2	24	1
3	6	1	2	0	310	0	4	20	1
3	4	1	1	0	320	0	2	20	1
4	9	2.5	0	0	10	0	4	14	2
5	11	2	0	0	90	4	6	12	2
5	11	1.5	0	0	15	2	8	10	2
4	10	2.5	0	0	25	2	6	16	2
5	10	1.5	0	0	270	2	4	13	2
0	0	0	0	0	80	0	0	0	0
0	0	0	0	0	40	0	0	23	0
0	0	0	0	0	35	0	0	24	0
0	0	0	0	0	55	0	0	40	0
0	0	0	0	0	0	0	0	44	0
0	0	0	0	0	0	0	0	37	0
0	0	0	0	0	55	0	0	48	0

Soft Drinks – Sole, cooked dry heat FOOD NAME	Portion Size	Calories	
Cream	12 oz	180	
Root Beer	12 oz	160	
Mountain Dew			
Amp	8 oz	110	
Baja Blast	8 oz	110	
Code Red	8 oz	110	
Livewire	8 oz	110	
MDX	8 oz	120	
Regular and caffeine-free	8 oz	110	
Pepsi			
Diet, all	8 oz	0	
Regular and caffeine free	8 oz	100	
Twist	8 oz	100	
Wild Cherry	8 oz	110	
Vanilla	8 oz	110	
Schweppes			
Club Soda	8 oz	0	
Ginger Ale	8 oz	80	
Ginger Ale, Diet	8 oz	0	
Ginger Ale, Diet, Grape	8 oz	0	
Tonic Water	8 oz	90	
Sierra Mist			
Free	8 oz	0	
Regular	8 oz	100	
SOLE, cooked dry heat	3 oz	99	

Protein (g)	Total Fat (g)	Sat. Fat (g)	Trans Fat (g)	Chol. (mg)	Sodium (mg)	Calcium (%)	Iron (%)	Carbs (g)	Fiber (g)
0	0	0	0	0	75	0	0	48	0
0	0	0	0	0	55	0	0	43	0
0	0	0	0	0	70	0	0	30	0
0	0	0	0	0	35	0	0	30	0
0	0	0	0	0	70	0	0	31	0
0	0	0	0	0	45	0	0	31	0
0	0	0	0	0	40	0	0	33	0
0	0	0	0	0	50	0	0	31	0
0	0	0	0	0	25	0	0	0	0
0	0	0	0	0	25	0	0	27	0
0	0	0	0	0	35	0	0	28	0
0	0	0	0	0	25	0	0	29	0
0	0	0	0	0	25	0	0	28	0
0	0	0	0	0	65	0	0	0	0
0	0	0	0	0	40	0	0	23	0
0	0	0	0	0	80	0	0	0	0
0	0	0	0	0	75	0	0	0	0
0	0	0	0	0	35	0	0	23	0
0	0	0	0	0	25	0	0	0	0
0	0	0	0	0	25	0	0	26	0
21	1	0	0	58	89	2	2	0	0

FOOD NAME	Portion Size	Calories	
SORBET			
Ben & Jerry's			
Berried Treasure	½ c	110	
Jamaican Me Crazy	½ c	130	
Strawberry Kiwi	½ c	110	
Häagen-Dazs			
Chocolate	½ c	130	
Mango	½ c	120	
Strawberry	½ c	120	
Tropical	½ c	150	
Zesty Lemon	½ c	110	
SOUPS—Canned			
Campbell's			
Bean w/ Bacon	½ c	170	
Beef Noodle	½ c	70	
Beef w/ Vegetables & Barley	½ c	90	
Black Bean	½ c	110	
Broccoli Cheese	½ c	100	
Chicken & Dumplings	½ c	80	
Chicken & Stars	½ c	70	
Chicken Gumbo	½ c	60	
Chicken Noodle	½ c	60	
Chicken Vegetable	½ c	80	
Chicken Won Ton	½ c	60	
Cream of Broccoli, 98% f-f	½ c	70	

Protein (g)	Total Fat (g)	Sat. Fat (g)	Trans Fat (g)	Chol (mg)	Sodium (mg)	Calcium (%)	Iron (%)	Carbs (g)	Fiber (g)
0	0	0	0	0	5	0	0	29	1
0	0	0	0	0	10	0	0	33	4
0	0	0	0	0	10	0	0	28	1
2	0.5	0	0	0	70	0	6	28	0
0	0	0	0	0	10	0	0	37	0
0	0	0	0	0	10	0	0	30	<1
0	0	0	0	0	25	0	0	38	0
0	0	0	0	0	25	2	0	28	0
8	4	1.5	0	5	860	6	10	26	8
4	2.5	0.5	0	15	870	0	4	9	<1
5	1.5	1	0	10	890	0	4	15	3
6	1.5	0.5	0	0	960	4	10	18	6
2	4.5	2	0	5	820	4	0	12	0
3	3	1	0	15	960	0	2	10	1
3	2	0.5	0	5	860	0	2	10	1
2	1	0.5	0	5	870	2	0	10	1
3	1.5	0.5	0	15	890	0	2	8	<1
3	1	0.5	0	5	890	2	2	15	2
4	1	0.5	0	10	870	0	2	8	0
2	2	0.5	0	<5	700	2	0	10	2

Soups—Canned

FOOD NAME	Portion Size	Calories	
Cream of Celery	½ c	90	
Cream of Chicken	½ c	120	
Cream of Chicken, 98% f-f	½ c	70	
Cream of Mushroom	½ c	100	
Cream of Potato	½ c	90	
Cream of Shrimp	½ c	90	
Creamy Tomato Ranchero	½ c	130	
Fiesta Chili Beef	½ c	170	
Fiesta Nacho Cheese	½ c	120	
French Onion	½ c	45	
Golden Mushroom	½ c	80	
Goldfish Meatball	½ c	80	
Green Pea	½ c	180	
Hearty Vegetable w/ Pasta	½ c	90	
Manhattan Clam Chowder	½ c	70	
Minestrone	½ c	90	
New England Clam Chowder	½ c	90	
New England Clam Chowder, 98% f-f	½ c	80	
Old Fashioned Vegetable	½ c	80	
Pepper Pot	½ c	90	
Scotch Broth	½ c	70	
Southwest Style Queso	½ c	150	
Split Pea w/ Ham & Bacon	½ c	180	
Tomato	½ c	90	
Tomato Noodle	½ c	120	

Protein (g)	Total Fat (g)	Sat. Fat (g)	Trans Fat (g)	Chol. (mg)	Sodium (mg)	Calcium (%)	Iron (%)	Carbs (g)	Fiber (g)
1	6	0.5	0	<5	860	2	0	9	3
3	8	2.5	0	10	870	0	0	10	2
2	2.5	1	0	10	790	0	0	10	1
1	6	1.5	0	5	870	0	0	9	2
2	2	1	0	5	800	0	2	15	2
1	6	2	0	15	880	2	0	8	1
3	6	2	0	5	800	2	2	16	4
7	5	2	0	10	770	4	8	25	8
3	8	3	0	10	790	8	0	10	1
2	1.5	1	0	<5	900	2	0	6	1
2	3.5	1	0	5	890	0	0	10	1
4	2.5	1.5	0	10	750	0	2	11	2
9	3	1	0	0	870	2	8	28	4
3	0.5	0	0	0	890	2	4	10	0
2	0.5	0.5	0	<5	880	2	4	12	2
4	1	0.5	0	<5	960	2	6	17	3
4	2.5	0.5	0	5	880	2	4	13	5
3	2	0.5	0	<5	940	0	2	13	1
3	1.5	0.5	0	5	920	2	2	14	5
5	4	1.5	0	25	980	2	4	9	1
3	2	1	0	5	880	0	2	9	2
4	7	2.5	0	10	810	4	2	18	4
10	3.5	2	0	5	850	2	8	27	5
2	0	0	0	0	710	0	4	20	1
3	0.5	0	0	5	660	0	0	25	2

Soups—Canned FOOD NAME	Portion Size	Calories	
Vegetable Beef	½ c	80	
Vegetarian Vegetable	½ c	90	
Campbell's Chunky			
Baked Potato w/ Cheddar & Bacon	1 c	160	
Baked Potato w/ Steak & Cheese	1 c	210	
Beef w/ Country Vegetable	1 c	150	
Cheese Tortellini w/ Chicken & Vegetables	1 c	110	
Chicken & Dumplings	1 c	180	
Chicken Mushroom Chowder	1 c	210	
Grilled Chicken & Sausage Gumbo	1 c	140	
Hearty Bean & Ham	1 c	180	
Hearty Beef Barley	1 c	170	
Honey Roasted Ham w/ Potatoes	1 c	130	
New England Clam Chowder	1 c	190	
Pepper Steak	1 c	120	
Savory Pot Roast	1 c	120	
Savory Vegetable	1c	110	
Split Pea & Ham	1 c	170	
Steak & Potato	1 c	130	
Tomato Cheese Ravioli w/ Vegetables	1 c	160	
Turkey pot pie	1 c	180	
Campbell's Chunky Microwaveable			
Beef w/ Country Vegetables	1 c	150	
Chicken & Dumplings	1 c	190	
New England Clam Chowder	1 c	200	

Protein (g)	Total Fat (g)	Sat. Fat (g)	Trans Fat (g)	Chol. (mg)	Sodium (mg)	Calcium (%)	Iron (%)	Carbs (g)	Fiber (g)
5	1	0.5	0	5	890	2	4	15	3
3	0.5	0	0	0	790	2	4	18	2
6	5	2.5	0	15	940	4	4	21	1
9	10	2.5	0	15	940	2	8	21	3
10	2.6	1	0	15	890	2	8	21	4
5	2	1	0	10	890	4	2	18	2
9	7	2	0	30	890	2	2	19	4
7	12	3	0	10	910	2	2	19	3
8	2.5	1	0	15	850	2	2	21	3
11	2	0.5	0	10	780	6	10	30	8
10	2.5	1	0	10	890	2	6	26	4
8	2.5	1	0	15	810	4	4	20	3
6	9	2	0	10	890	2	4	21	2
8	1.5	0.5	0	15	800	2	6	18	3
8	1.5	1	0	15	880	2	4	18	3
3	1	0.5	0	0	770	4	4	22	4
12	2.5	1	0	10	780	2	8	27	4
10	2	0.5	0	15	920	0	6	18	2
5	3	2	0	5	920	6	4	27	3
9	7	2	0	20	870	2	2	20	4
10	3	1.5	0	20	900	2	4	21	5
10	9	2	0	40	890	2	0	18	3
6	12	2.5	0	15	870	8	10	18	3

FOOD NAME	Portion Size	Calories	
Sirloin Burger w/ Country Vegetables	1 c	160	
Campbell's Healthy Choice			
Bean & Ham	1 c	170	
Chunky Beef & Potato	1 c	110	
Fiesta Chicken	1 c	100	
Garden Vegetable	1 c	120	
New England Clam Chowder	1 c	110	
Roasted Chicken w/ Garlic	1 c	120	
Split Pea & Ham	1 c	170	
Vegetable Beef	1 c	130	
Zesty Gumbo	1 c	100	
Campbell's Healthy Request			
Chicken Noodle	½ c	60	
Cream of Celery	½ c	70	
Cream of Mushroom	½ c	70	
Minestrone	½ c	80	
Vegetable Beef	½ c	90	
Campbell's Select			
Beef w/ Roasted Barley	1 c	130	
Chicken Vegetable Medley	1 c	110	
Creamy Chicken Alfredo	1 c	180	
Fiesta Vegetable	1 c	120	
Italian Style Wedding	1 c	110	
Minestrone	1 c	100	
New England Clam Chowder, 98% f-f	1 c	110	

Protein (g)	Total Fat (g)	Sat. Fat (g)	Trans Fat (g)	Chol. (mg)	Sodium (mg)	Calcium (%)	Iron (%)	Carbs (g)	Fiber (g)
10	4	2	0	15	870	2	6	18	4
11	2.5	1	0	10	480	8	15	29	6
8	1	0	0	10	480	0	6	19	2
6	2	0.5	0	5	480	4	4	17	3
6	1	0	0	0	480	4	10	25	4
4	1.5	1	0	15	480	2	6	21	3
8	2	0	0	5	480	2	2	21	2
11	2.5	1	0	5	480	2	6	30	4
9	1	0	0	10	480	4	10	24	4
6	2	1	0	20	480	4	6	16	3
3	2	0.5	0	10	450	0	0	8	1
1	2	0.5	0	<5	430	10	0	12	1
1	1	0.5	0	<5	470	10	0	10	1
3	0.5	0	0	5	460	4	6	15	3
5	1	0.5	0	5	480	2	4	15	3
9	1	0.5	0	10	920	2	4	22	2
7	0.5	0.5	0	10	870	2	0	19	2
10	7	1	0	10	930	4	4	18	2
4	0.5	0	0	0	840	4	4	24	4
7	2.5	2	0	10	840	4	4	16	2
5	0.5	0	0	0	950	4	6	20	3
5	1.5	0	0	10	850	2	4	18	2

Soups—Canned

FOOD NAME	Portion Size	Calories
Potato Broccoli Cheese	1 c	120
Roasted Beef Tips	1 c	120
Roasted Chicken w/ Rotini	1 c	100
Savory Lentil	1 c	140
Split Pea w/ Roasted Ham	1 c	160
Tomato Garden	1 c	100
Vegetable Medley	1 c	100
Campbell's Soup at Hand		
Blended Vegetable Medley	1 cont	100
Chicken & Stars	1 cont	60
Cream of Broccoli	1 cont	150
Mexican Style Fiesta	1 cont	150
Pizza	1 cont	140
Velvety Potato	1 cont	160
Imagine		
Crab Bisque	1 c	130
Lobster Bisque	1 c	130
Organic Creamy Broccoli	1 c	60
Organic Creamy Butternut Squash	1 c	90
Organic Creamy Chicken	1 c	70
Organic Creamy Sweet Corn	1 c	120
Organic Creamy Sweet Potato	1 c	110
Organic Creamy Tomato Basil	1 c	90
Lipton Cup of Soup		
Asian Beef Noodle	1 pkt	70

Protein (g)	Total Fat (g)	Sat. Fat (g)	Trans Fat (g)	Chol. (mg)	Sodium (mg)	Calcium (%)	Iron (%)	Carbs (g)	Fiber (g)
3	4	1	0	<5	890	4	2	18	4
9	1.5	0.5	0	15	890	4	2	18	4
8	0.5	0.5	0	10	860	2	0	16	2
8	0.5	0.5	0	5	860	2	20	27	6
10	1	0	0	5	830	4	8	29	5
3	0.5	0.5	0	5	700	1	1	21	2
3	0.5	0	0	0	900	4	4	21	3
3	1.5	0.5	0	<5	890	2	0	19	4
3	1.5	0.5	0	5	890	0	2	10	2
3	7	2	0	5	890	2	4	17	7
6	5	2.5	0	15	990	2	8	21	3
6	1	0.5	0	15	880	8	4	27	2
2	7	1	0	<5	870	2	2	21	4
5	5	3	0	16	690	15	2	16	0
5	5	3	0	15	690	15	2	15	0
3	1.5	0	0	0	470	2	4	10	2
0	2	0	0	0	460	4	4	18	2
3	1.5	0	0	5	680	2	2	12	1
4	3	0.5	0	0	450	2	4	20	3
2	1.5	0	0	0	400	2	4	23	
3	1.5	0	0	0	430	4	4	17	2
1	'	0	0	0	580	0	2	14	0

Soups—Canned FOOD NAME	Portion Size	Calories	
Broccoli Cheese	1 pkt	90	
Chicken Noodle	1 pkt	80	
Cream of Chicken	1 pkt	70	
Spring Vegetable	1 pkt	1	
Tomato w/ Croutons	1 pkt	90	
Progresso—50% Less Sodium			
Chicken Gumbo	1 c	110	
Chicken Noodle	1 c	90	
Garden Vegetable	1 c	100	
Minestrone	1 c	120	
Progresso—Rich & Hearty			
Beef Barley Vegetable	1 c	130	
Chicken Corn Chowder	1 c	210	
Chicken & Homestyle Noodles	1 c	110	
Chicken Pot Pie style	1 c	170	
New England Clam Chowder	1 c	190	
Sirloin Steak & Vegetables	1 c	130	
Steak & Homestyle Noodles	1 c	120	
Steak & Sautéed Mushrooms	1 c	110	
Progresso—Traditional			
Beef & Baked Potato	1 c	100	
Beef Barley	1 c	140	
Beef Barley, 98% f-f	1 c	120	
Beef & Mushroom	1 c	100	
Beef & Vegetables	1 c	100	

Protein (g)	Total Fat (g)	Sat. Fat (g)	Trans Fat (g)	Chol. (mg)	Sodium (mg)	Calcium (%)	Iron (%)	Carbs (g)	Fiber (g)
2	1.5	1	0	5	840	4	0	17	0
2	0.5	0	0	<5	920	0	0	17	0
1	1.5	0	0	0	730	0	0	14	0
0	0	0	0	0	720	0	4	11	<1
1	2.5	0	0	0	870	0	0	16	1
7	1.5	0.5	0	15	450	2	4	18	2
7	1.5	0	0	20	470	2	4	12	1
3	0	0	0	0	450	4	6	12	1
5	2	0.5	0	0	470	4	6	24	4
9	1	0.5	0	15	970	2	6	22	3
7	9	2.5	0	1.5	790	2	4	23	2
8	2	0.5	0	25	920	2	4	14	1
8	6	1.5	0	15	940	2	4	21	2
6	9	2	0	10	840	2	6	22	2
8	2	1	0	15	870	2	6	21	2
9	3	1	0	25	830	1	0	6	4
7	2	0.5	0	10	930	0	6	18	1
6	2.5	1	0	15	930	2	4	15	1
9	3.5	1.5	0	15	650	2	6	18	2
7	1.5	0.5	0	10	720	2	6	20	4
7	0.5	0	0	15	06-	2	6	13	1
7	1	0	0	15	850	4	6	17	2

Soups—Canned

FOOD NAME	Portion Size	Calories	
Chickaria	1 c	130	
Chicken & Barley	1 c	100	
Chicken Cheese Enchilada, Carb Monitor	1 c	170	
Chicken Noodle	1 c	100	
Chicken Noodle, 99% f-f	1 c	100	
Chicken & Rotini	1 c	100	
Chicken Sausage Gumbo	1 c	130	
Chicken Vegetable, Carb Monitor	1 c	70	
Chicken & Wild Rice	1 c	100	
Homestyle Chicken	1 c	100	
Italian style Wedding	1 c	130	
New England Clam Chowder	1 c	190	
New England Clam Chowder, 99% f-f	1 c	120	
Split Pea w/ Ham	1 c	150	
Turkey Noodle	1 c	80	
Tuscan Meatball, Carb Monitor	1 c	100	
Progresso—Vegetable Classics			
Creamy Mushroom	1 c	130	
French Onion	1 c	50	
Garden Vegetable	1 c	90	
Lentil	1 c	150	
Minestrone	1 c	110	
Tomato Basil	1 c	160	
Vegetable	1 c	80	
Vegetable Italiano	1 c	100	

Protein (g)	Total Fat (g)	Sat. Fat (g)	Trans Fat (g)	Chol. (mg)	Sodium (mg)	Calcium (%)	Iron (%)	Carbs (g)	Fiber (g)
8	5	1.5	0	15	920	2	6	12	<1
6	2.5	0.5	0	25	900	0	4	16	3
8	12	4	0	25	970	6	2	8	<1
7	2.5	0.5	0	25	950	2	4	12	1
6	2	0.5	0	20	950	2	4	12	1
7	2	0.5	0	15	960	2	2	13	1
6	4	1.5	0	15	900	2	4	18	1
6	2	1	0	20	840	2	2	7	1
6	1.5	0.5	0	15	870	2	2	15	1
6	2	0	0	10	800	0	4	14	1
6	5	2	0	15	940	4	6	15	1
6	10	2.5	0	10	890	2	6	20	2
5	2	0	0	5	720	0	6	21	2
9	1	0.5	0	10	730	2	6	25	4
5	1.5	0	0	15	930	0	4	12	1
5	5	2.5	0	15	840	6	6	9	1
2	10	3	0	10	820	0	0	9	1
1	1.5	0.5	0	<5	850	2	2	8	<1
3	0	0	0	0	940	0	4	20	3
9	2	0.5	0	0	870	4	15	28	5
4	2	0.5	0	0	980	4	8	19	0
2	3	0.5	0	0	960	2	6	30	1
3	0.5	0	0	0	950	2	4	16	2
2	2	0.5	0	0	1050	2	2	18	3

Soups—Canned – Sour Cream FOOD NAME	Portion Size	Calories	
Vegetarian Vegetable w/ Barley	1 c	100	
Top Ramen			
Beef	½ pkg	190	
Cajun Chicken	½ pkg	180	
Chicken	½ pkg	190	
Chicken Vegetable	½ pkg	190	
Oriental	½ pkg	190	
Shrimp	½ pkg	190	
Westbrae Natural			
Alabama Black Bean Gumbo	1 c	140	
Hearty Milano Minestrone	1 c	120	
Mediterranean Lentil	1 c	140	
Old World Split Pea	1 c	150	
Santa Fe Vegetable	1 c	160	
Tuscany Tomato	¾ c	70	
SOUR CREAM			
Breakstone's			
All Natural	2 Tbs	60	
Fat-free	2 Tbs	30	
Reduced Fat	2 Tbs	40	
Daisy			
Light	2 Tbs	40	
No Fat	2 Tbs	20	
Regular	2 Tbs	60	
Knudsen			

Protein (g)	Total Fat (g)	Sat. Fat (g)	Trans Fat (g)	Chol. (mg)	Sodium (mg)	Calcium (%)	Iron (%)	Carbs (g)	Fiber (g)
3	0.5	0	0	0	980	2	6	20	4
5	7	3.5	0	0	760	0	15	27	2
5	7	3.5	0	0	1020	0	10	26	1
5	7	3.5	0	0	910	0	10	26	2
5	7	4	0	0	830	0	15	26	1
5	7	3.5	0	0	800	0	10	26	1
5	7	3.5	0	0	860	0	15	26	1
8	0	0	0	0	530	6	10	26	6
7	0	0	0	0	570	8	10	24	6
10	0	0	0	0	540	4	20	24	10
10	0	0	0	0	590	2	15	28	6
9	0	0	0	0	380	6	15	31	8
2	0	0	0	0	710	2	8	16	0
1	5	3.5	0	20	10	2	0	1	0
1	0	0	0	5	25	4	0	5	0
1	3	2	0	15	20	6	0	2	0
2	2.5	2	0	25	25	4	0	2	0
2	0	0	0	0	15	4	0	1	0
1	5	3.5	0	20	15	2	0	1	0

FOOD NAME	Portion Size	Calories	
Fat-free	2 Tbs	30	
Hampshire	2 Tbs	60	
Light	2 Tbs	30	
SOY BEVERAGES			
Edensoy			
Carob, organic	8 oz	170	
Chocolate, organic	8 oz	180	
Extra original	8 oz	130	
Extra Vanilla	8 oz	150	
Light, original	8 oz	100	
Light, Vanilla	8 oz	110	
Original	8 oz	140	
Vanilla	8 oz	150	
Pacific			
Organic soy, plain, low fat	8 oz	70	
Organic soy, vanilla, low fat	8 oz	80	
Organic soy, ultra, plain	8 oz	120	
Organic soy, ultra, vanilla	8 oz	130	
Silk			
Chai	8 oz	130	
Chocolate	8 oz	140	
Enhanced	8 oz	110	
Light Chocolate	8 oz	120	
Light Vanilla	8 oz	80	
Mocha	8 oz	140	

Protein (g)	Total Fat (g)	Sat. Fat (g)	Trans Fat (g)	Chol. (mg)	Sodium (mg)	Calcium (%)	Iron (%)	Carbs (g)	Fiber (g)
2	0	0	0	5	25	6	0	5	0
1	6	3.5	0	20	10	2	0	1	0
2	2	1	0	10	20	4	0	2	0
7	4	0.5	0	0	95	8	8	28	<1
8	4	1	0	0	105	10	10	28	<1
11	4	0.5	0	0	100	20	10	13	<1
7	3	0	0	0	90	20	6	23	<1
5	2	0	0	0	90	10	4	15	0
4	1	0	0	0	110	10	4	22	0
11	5	0.5	0	0	105	10	10	14	<1
7	3	0.5	0	0	85	8	6	24	<1
5	2.5	0	0	0	115	2	4	9	1
5	2.5	0	0	0	115	2	4	9	<1
10	4	0.5	0	0	150	50	10	12	1
10	4	0.5	0	0	150	50	10	14	1
6	3.5	0.5	0	0	100	30	6	19	0
5	3.5	0.5	0	0	100	30	8	23	2
7	5	0.5	0	0	120	35	6	8	1
5	1.5	0	0	0	100	30	8	22	2
6	2	0	0	0	95	30	6	10	1
5	3.5	0.5	0	0	100	30	6	22	0

FOOD NAME	Portion Size	Calories
Plain	8 oz	100
Silk Live! Blueberry	1 cont	230
Silk Live! Mango	1 cont	230
Silk Live! Peach	1 cont	220
Silk Live! Strawberry	1 cont	220
Vanilla	8 oz	100
Very Vanilla	8 oz	130
SOY SAUCE—See "Sauces"		
SOYBEANS (also see "Tofu")		
Cascadian Farm, Edamame	⅔ c	120
Fresh, cooked, no salt	1 c	298
Roasted, no salt	1 oz	133
SOY SNACKS		
Hain, Caramel	7 pcs	40
Hain, Ranch	9 pcs	60
Hain, White Cheddar Munchies	9 pcs	60
SPAGHETTI—See "Pasta"		
SPAGHETTI SQUASH, cooked, no salt	1 c	42
SPINACH		
Fresh, cooked, drained	1 c	41
Fresh, raw	1 c	7
Birds Eye, chopped or leaf, frozen	⅓ c	30
Birds Eye, creamed w/ real cream	½ c	100
Green Giant, frozen, no sauce	½ c	25
Green Giant, frozen, creamed	½ c	70

Protein (g)	Total Fat (g)	Sat. Fat (g)	Trans Fat (g)	Chol. (mg)	Sodium (mg)	Calcium (%)	Iron (%)	Carbs (g)	Fiber (g)
7	4	0.5	0	0	120	30	6	8	1
7	4	0.5	0	0	120	35	10	42	3
7	4	0.5	0	0	120	35	10	41	3
7	4	0.5	0	0	120	35	10	38	3
7	4	0.5	0	0	120	35	10	40	3
6	3.5	0.5	0	0	95	30	6	10	1
6	4	0.5	0	0	140	35	6	19	1
10	5	0.5	0	0	10	10	10	9	3
29	15	2	0	0	2	18	49	17	10
10	7	1	0	0	1	4	6	9	5
2	0	0	0	0	10	20	2	8	<1
3	2	0	0	0	150	30	4	8	0
3	2.5	0.5	0	0	240	30	4	6	1
1	0	0	0	0	28	3	3	10	2
5	0	0	0	0	126	24	36	7	4
1	0	0	0	0	24	3	5	1	1
2	0	0	0	0	125	8	4	3	1
3	7	3	0	35	630	10	4	7	1
2	0	0	0	0	200	6	4	3	1
3	2.5	1	0.5	0	520	10	2	9	1

FOOD NAME	Portion Size	Calories
Green Giant, frozen, cut leaf/butter	½ c	30
S&W, canned, leaf	½ c	30
SQUASH—See specific types		
STRAWBERRIES, fresh raw	1 c	49
Cascadian Farm, frozen	1 c	45
STUFFING		·
Pepperidge Farm		
Corn Bread	¾ c	170
Country Style	¾ c	140
Cube	¾ c	140
One Step Chicken	½ c	160
One Step Turkey	½ c	170
Sage & Onion	¾ c	140
Stove Top		
Chicken	⅙ box	110
Chicken, lower sodium	⅙ box	110
Chicken w/ whole wheat	⅕ box	100
Cornbread One Step	⅛ box	120
Homestyle Herb One Step	⅛ box	110
Pork	⅙ box	110
Turkey	⅙ box	110
SUGAR		
Brown	1 tsp	11
Powdered	1 tsp	10
White, granulated	1 tsp	15

Protein (g)	Total Fat (g)	Sat. Fat (g)	Trans Fat (g)	Chol. (mg)	Sodium (mg)	Calcium (%)	Iron (%)	Carbs (g)	Fiber (g)
2	1	0	0	<5	330	8	4	4	2
2	0	0	0	0	360	10	6	4	2
1	0	0	0	0	2	2	4	12	3
<1	0	0	0	0	0	2	4	13	3
4	2	0	0	0	480	4	10	33	2
5	1	0	0	0	380	0	8	27	2
4	1	0	0	0	530	4	10	28	2
2	4	1	0	0	520	2	8	25	2
4	7	1	0	0	540	2	6	23	1
5	1	0	0	0	540	8	10	20	0
4	1	0	0	0	430	0	6	20	1
4	1	0	0	0	260	0	6	21	1
5	1.5	0	0	0	480	0	8	18	3
3	3	0	0	0	530	0	4	19	1
3	2.5	0	0	0	440	0	6	19	1
3	1	0	0	0	450	0	6	20	1
3	1	0	0	0	460	0	6	20	1
0	0	0	0	0	1	0	0	3	0
0	0	0	0	0	0	0	0	2	0
0	0	0	0	0	0	0	0	4	0

FOOD NAME	Portion Size	Calories
SUNFLOWER SEEDS, dried	1 oz	161
Planters, dry roasted	1 oz	180
SWEET POTATOES		
Baked in Skin w/ salt	1 med	103
Green Giant Candied, frozen	¾ c	240
Green Giant, Sweet Potato		
Casserole, frozen	1c	200
McCain Sweet Potato Fry	3 oz	120
SWORDFISH, cooked, dry heat	3 oz	132
TACO SHELLS		
Old El Paso	3	150
Taco Bell	3	150
TANGERINE, raw	1 c	103
Minute Maid Orange Tangerine Juice	8 oz	110
Noble, Tangerine Juice	8 oz	125
POM, Tangerine Juice	8 oz	140
TEA		
Celestial Seasonings		
All Herbal, Dessert, Holiday, Black teas	1 bag	0
Cinnamon Spice Teahouse Chai	3 Tbs	110
Sweet Coconut Thai Chai	3 Tbs	110
Vanilla Ginger Chai	3 Tbs	110
Lipton		
Chailatta, original	3 Tbs	120
Chailatta, Vanilla	3 Tbs	120

Protein (g)	Total Fat (g)	Sat. Fat (g)	Trans Fat (g)	Chol. (mg)	Sodium (mg)	Calcium (%)	Iron (%)	Carbs (g)	Fiber (g)
6	14	1	0	0	1	3	11	5	3
7	15	1.5	0	0	260	4	10	6	3
2	0	0	0	0	280	4	4	24	4
2	7	1	1.5	0	430	2	4	41	3
3	10	1.5	1.5	0	420	2	4	28	3
0	3	0.5	0	0	180	2	2	22	2
22	4	1	0	43	98	1	5	0	0
2	7	1.5	2.5	0	135	2	0	20	0
2	6	1	0	0	5	0	0	22	2
2	1	0	0	0	4	7	2	20	4
2	0	0	0	0	15	35	0	27	0
1	0	0	0	0	0	0	0	30	0
<1	0	0	0	0	20	2	0	34	0
0	0	0	0	0	0	0	0	0	0
2	0	0	0	0	80	15	0	25	0
2	0	0	0	0	75	10	0	25	0
2	0	0	0	0	80	15	0	25	0
3	2	0	0	<5	180	8	0	21	0
3	2	0	0	<5	200	8	0	19	0

Tea – Tofu FOOD NAME	Portion Size	Calories	
Hot tea, Black or Green	1 bag	0	
Iced Green Tea w/ Citrus	8 oz	80	
Iced Tea Mix, Sweetened, Lemon	4 tsp	70	
Iced Tea Mix, Sweetened, Raspberry	1.5 Tbs	80	
Original Iced Tea, bottles	8 oz	70	
White Tea w/ Tangerine, bottles	8 oz	60	
TEMPEH			
Lightlife, Organic Flax	4 oz	220	
Lightlife, Organic Garden Veggie	4 oz	200	
Lightlife Organic, Three Grain	4 oz	230	
Lightlife Organic, Wild Rice	4 oz	230	
TOFU			
Fresh Tofu Inc.			
Baked Stuffed	1 pc	160	
Organic Baked	2 oz	90	
Mori-Nu			
Chinese Spice Seasoned	3 oz	50	
Enriched Silken, firm	3 oz	70	
Japanese Miso Seasoned	3 oz	60	
Silken, extra firm	3 oz	48	
Silken, lite extra firm	3 oz	35	
Silken, soft	3 oz	45	
Nasoya			
Chinese Spice Firm	¼ pkg	90	
Extra Firm	⅕ pkg	80	

Protein (g)	Total Fat (g)	Sat. Fat (g)	Trans Fat (g)	Chol. (mg)	Sodium (mg)	Calcium (%)	Iron (%)	Carbs (g)	Fiber (g)
0	0	0	0	0	0	0	0	0	0
0	0	0	0	0	0	0	0	21	0
0	0	0	0	0	0	0	0	18	0
0	0	0	0	0	0	0	0	19	0
0	0	0	0	0	5	0	0	18	0
0	0	0	0	0	5	0	0	16	0
21	9	1.5	0	0	0	0	0	16	30
22	10	1.5	0	0	220	0	0	17	14
18	9	1.5	0	0	0	0	0	21	8
19	7	1	0	0	5	0	0	22	12
17	4.5	0.5	0	0	260	0	15	14	6
9	6	1	0	0	260	4	10	1	0
6	2	0	0	0	240	4	6	3	0
6	2.5	0	0	0	40	10	4	60	0
7	2.5	0	0	0	240	4	6	3	0
6	1.5	0	0	0	55	2	4	2	0
6	0.5	0	0	0	85	4	4	1	0
4	2.5	0	0	0	0	2	4	2	0
8	5	1	0	0	220	4	6	3	1
8	4	0.5	0	0	0	6	8	2	1

Tofu – Tomatoes FOOD NAME	Portion Size	Calories	
Garlic & Onion	¼ pkg	90	
Lite Firm	¼ pkg	40	
Silken	⅕ pkg	45	
Soft	⅕ pkg	60	
TOMATOES			
Fresh, Red, cooked	1 c	43	
Fresh, Red Cherry	1 c	31	
Fresh, Red	1 med	26	
Fresh, Red Plum	1	13	
Fresh, Yellow, Chopped	1 c	21	
Canned			
Del Monte, diced w/ Garlic & Onion	½ c	40	
Del Monte, diced Pasta Style	½ c	45	
Del Monte, stewed, Mexican	½ c	35	
Del Monte, wedges	½ c	35	
Eden Organic, crushed w/ Basil	¼ c	20	
Eden Organic, diced w/ Green Chilis	½ c	30	
Eden Organic, whole	½ c	30	
Muir Glen, crushed w/ Basil	¼ c	25	
Muir Glen, diced w/ Italian Herbs	½ c	30	
Muir Glen, whole, Fire Roasted	½ c	25	
Muir Glen, whole, Peeled Plum	½ c	25	
Progresso, crushed	¼ c	20	
Progresso, diced	½ c	25	
Progresso, whole peeled w/ Basil	½ c	20	

Protein (g)	Total Fat (g)	Sat. Fat (g)	Trans Fat (g)	Chol. (mg)	Sodium (mg)	Calcium (%)	Iron (%)	Carbs (g)	Fiber (g)
8	5	1	0	0	250	4	6	3	1
7	1.5	0	0	0	25	15	8	1	<1
4	2	0	0	0	0	6	4	1	0
6	3	1	0	0	0	10	6	1	<1
2	0	0	0	0	28	3	9	10	2
1	0	0	0	0	13	1	4	7	2
1	0	0	0	0	11	1	3	6	1
1	0	0	0	0	6	0	2	3	1
1	0	0	0	0	32	2	4	4	1
2	0.5	0	0	0	610	2	10	8	<1
1	0	0	0	0	560	2	2	11	2
1	0	0	0	0	400	2	2	9	2
1	0	0	0	0	380	2	2	9	2
1	0	0	0	0	0	2	4	3	1
2	0	0	0	0	35	2	2	5	2
1	0	0	0	0	10	0	4	4	1
1	0	0	0	0	190	0	2	5	1
1	0	0	0	0	350	2	4	6	1
1	0	0	0	0	260	2	4	5	1
1	0	0	0	0	260	2	4	5	1
<1	0	0	0	0	95	2	4	3	0
1	0	0	0	0	250	2	4	5	1
1	0	0	0	0	260	2	4	4	1

Tomato Juice – Toppings, Dessert FOOD NAME	Portion Size	Calories	
TOMATO JUICE			
Campbell's, Healthy Request	8 oz	50	
Campbell's, original	8 oz	50	
Del Monte	8 oz	50	
TOMATO PASTE/PUREE			
Hunt's, paste	2 Tbs	25	
Hunt's, paste, no salt	2 Tbs	30	
Hunt's, paste, w/ Basil, Garlic, Oregano	2 Tbs	25	
Hunt's, purée	4 oz	30	
Muir Glen, paste	2 Tbs	25	
Muir Glen, purée	¼ c	25	
S&W, paste	2 Tbs	30	
S&W, purée	¼ c	30	
TOPPINGS, DESSERT			
Cool Whip, Chocolate	2 Tbs	25	
Cool Whip, French Vanilla	2 Tbs	25	
Cool Whip, lite	2 Tbs	20	
Cool Whip, regular	2 Tbs	25	
Cool Whip, sugar free	2 Tbs	20	
Smucker's, Butterscotch Caramel	2 Tbs	130	
Smucker's, Dove Dark Chocolate	2 Tbs	140	
Smucker's, Plate Scrapers Caramel	2 Tbs	100	
Smucker's, Plate Scrapers Raspberry	2 Tbs	100	
Smucker's, Plate Scrapers Vanilla	2 Tbs	110	
Smucker's, Special Recipe Hot Fudge	2 Tbs	140	

Protein (g)	Total Fat (g)	Sat. Fat (g)	Trans Fat (g)	Chol. (mg)	Sodium (mg)	Calcium (%)	Iron (%)	Carbs (g)	Fiber (g)
2	0	0	0	0	480	2	0	10	2
2	0	0	0	0	680	2	2	10	2
2	0	0	0	0	760	4	10	10	1
1	0	0	0	0	00	0	2	6	2
1	0	0	0	0	15	0	0	6	2
2	0	0	0	0	260	0	4	6	2
1	0	0	0	0	450	6	2	7	2
1	0	0	0	0	90	0	2	6	2
1	0	0	0	0	30	0	4	6	1
2	0	0	0	0	20	0	4	6	1
1	0	0	0	0	15	0	4	2	2
0	1.5	1.5	0	0	0	0	0	2	0
0	1.5	1.5	0	0	0	0	0	2	0
0	1	1	0	0	0	0	0	3	0
0	1.5	1.5	0	0	0	0	0	2	0
0	1	1	0	0	0	0	0	3	0
1	1.	0.5	0	<5	70	4	0	30	<1
>1	5	1.5	0	0	80	0	6	22	1
1	0	0	0	0	105	0	0	25	0
0	0	0	0	0	5	0	0	25	0
1	1	0	0	0	0	0	0	24	0
2	4	1	0	0	70	6	4	22	<1

Tuna – Veal FOOD NAME	Portion Size	Calories	
TUNA			
Chicken of the Sea			
Chunk, lite in oil	2 oz	110	
Chunk lite in water	2 oz	60	
Chunk white in water	2 oz	60	
Genova Tonno in olive oil	2 oz	130	
Premium, Albacore, pouch	2 oz	60	
Solid white Albacore, in oil	2 oz	90	
Solid white Albacore in water	2 oz	70	
Yellowfin solid light, water	2 oz	70	
Starkist			
Chunk Light pouch	3 oz	90	
Chunk Light water, can	2 oz	60	
Gourmet Choice Fillet, water	2 oz	60	
Solid White Albacore, water	2 oz	70	
TURKEY			
Dark meat, roasted	1 oz	53	
Light meat, roasted	1 oz	44	
Louis Rich, breast & white	1 oz	28	
Louis Rich, pure ground	4 oz	190	
Louis Rich, smoked white, 95% f-f	1 oz	30	
TURNIP, cooked, no salt	1 c	34	
VEAL			
Breast, boneless, lean	3 oz	185	
Leg, lean	3 oz	128	

Protein (g)	Total Fat (g)	Sat. Fat (g)	Trans Fat (g)	Chol. (mg)	Sodium (mg)	Calcium (%)	Iron (%)	Carbs (g)	Fiber (g)
13	6	1	0	30	250	0	2	0	0
13	0.5	0	0	30	250	0	2	0	0
13	1	0	0	25	250	0	0	0	0
14	8	1	0	30	250	0	2	0	0
13	1	0	0	25	250	0	0	0	0
14	3	1	0	25	250	0	0	0	0
15	1	0	0	25	250	0	0	0	0
15	1	0	0	30	250	0	2	0	0
19	1	0	0	45	380	0	0	0	0
13	0.5	0	0	30	250	0	0	0	0
13	1	0	0	30	260	0	0	0	0
15	1	0	0	25	250	0	0	0	0
8	2	1	0	24	22	1	4	0	0
8	1	0	0	19	19	1	2	0	0
5	1	0	0	11	270	0	2	1	0
20	12	3.5	0	90	140	0	0	0	0
4	1	0	0	10	320	0	0	1	0
1	0	0	0	0	25	5	2	8	3
26	8	3	0	99	58	1	4	0	0
24	3	1	0	88	58	1	4	0	0

FOOD NAME	Portion Size	Calories	
Loin, lean	3 oz	149	
Rib, lean	3 oz	185	
Sirloin, lean	3 oz	143	
VEGETABLE JUICE			
Knudsen, Very Veggie, low sodium	8 oz	50	
Knudsen, Very Veggie, original	8 oz	50	
Knudsen, Very Veggie, spicy	8 oz	50	
V-8, calcium enriched	8 oz	50	
V-8, low sodium	8 oz	50	
V-8, picante	8 oz	50	
V-8, 100%	8 oz	50	
VEGETABLES, Mixed			
Canned			
Del Monte, Homestyle medley	½ c	70	
Del Monte Mixed	½ c	40	
Del Monte Mixed w/ Potatoes	½ c	45	
S&W Mixed	½ c	45	
Birds Eye			
Asian in Sesame Ginger	1 c	60	
Baby Corn & Vegetable Blend	⅔ c	50	
Baby Pea & Vegetable Blend	¾ c	40	
Baby Potato & Vegetable Blend	¾ c	40	
California Blend & Cheddar Cheese	½ c	80	
Classic Mixed	⅔ c	60	
Szechuan in Sesame Sauce	1 c	60	

Protein (g)	Total Fat (g)	Sat. Fat (g)	Trans Fat (g)	Chol. (mg)	Sodium (mg)	Calcium (%)	Iron (%)	Carbs (g)	Fiber (g)
22	6	2	0	90	82	2	4	0	0
29	7	2	0	122	84	2	7	0	0
22	5	2	0	88	72	1	4	0	0
2	0	0	0	0	35	2	4	11	2
2	0	0	0	0	580	2	4	11	2
2	0	0	0	0	590	2	4	11	2
2	0	0	0	0	460	30	4	11	2
2	0	0	0	0	140	2	2	10	2
2	0	0	0	0	590	4	2	10	2
2	0	0	0	0	590	4	4	10	2
1	2.5	0	0	0	380	4	2	11	2
2	0	0	0	0	360	2	4	8	2
2	0	0	0	0	360	4	4	10	2
2	0	0	0	0	360	4	4	10	2
2	1	0	0	0	630	2	2	12	2
2	1	0	0	0	10	2	2	9	3
2	0	0	0	0	20	2	2	7	2
1	0	0	0	0	20	2	2	8	1
2	4	2	0	5	390	6	2	8	1
2	0	0	0	0	20	2	2	12	2
1	2	0	0	0	460	2	2	9	2

FOOD NAME	Portion Size	Calories	
Tuscan Vegetables in Herbed Tomato	1 c	50	
Cascadian Farm			
California Style Blend	⅔ c	25	
Chinese Stir Fry	1 c	25	
Garden's Blend	¾ c	50	
Thai Stir Fry	¾ c	25	
Green Giant			
Baby Vegetable Medley	¾ c	40	
Boxed Alfredo	¾ c	60	
Garden Medley, prep	½ c	70	
Plain Mixed, prep	½ c	50	
Simply Steam Garden Medley, prep	½ c	50	
Szechuan Vegetables	¾ c	50	
Teriyaki Vegetables	1¼ c	70	
VINEGAR			
Eden Foods, Apple Cider or Red			
Wine, organic	1 Tbs	0	
Eden Foods, Brown Rice, organic	1 Tbs	2	
Eden Foods, Ume Plum, imported	1 tsp	0	
Progresso, Balsamic	1 Tbs	10	
WAFFLES—See "Frozen Breakfast";			
"Pancakes & Waffles"			
WALNUTS, Black, dried	1 oz	175	
Planters, Walnuts	1 oz	210	
WATERMELON, balls	1 c	46	

Protein (g)	Total Fat (g)	Sat. Fat (g)	Trans Fat (g)	Chol. (mg)	Sodium (mg)	Calcium (%)	Iron (%)	Carbs (g)	Fiber (g)
1	2	0	0	0	180	2	2	7	2
1	0	0	0	0	25	2	0	5	2
2	0	0	0	0	15	2	2	6	2
2	0	0	0	0	35	2	4	11	3
1	0	0	0	0	16	2	2	5	2
1	1	0	0	<5	250	2	2	9	2
3	2	1	0	5	420	6	2	10	3
2	0.5	0	0	0	220	2	4	14	2
2	0	0	0	0	40	0	2	11	2
2	0.5	0	0	0	280	2	4	11	1
2	0.5	0	0	0	410	2	2	9	2
2	4.5	1	1	0	490	2	2	7	2
0	0	0	0	0	0	0	0	0	0
0	0	0	0	0	0	0	0	0	0
0	0	0	0	0	1050	0	0	0	0
0	0	0	0	0	0	0	0	2	0
7	17	1	0	0	1	2	5	3	2
5	20	2	0	0	0	2	4	6	2
1	0	0	0	0	2	1	2	12	1

FOOD NAME	Portion Size	Calories	
WHITEFISH, cooked	3 oz	146	
Smoked	3 oz	92	
WINE, Red Table (average values)	5 oz	125	
Rose Table (average values)	3 oz	73	
White Table (average values)	5 oz	122	
YAM, boiled or baked, no salt, cubes	1 c	158	
Canned, candied (S&W)	½ c	170	
YOGURT			
Columbo			
Classic Banana Strawberry	8 oz	230	
Classic Blueberry, Cherry, Peach,			
Raspberry, Strawberry	8 oz	220	
Classic Vanilla	8 oz	190	
Light: Blueberry, Cherry Vanilla, Key			
Lime, Mixed Berry, Peach, Raspberry,			
Strawberry	8 oz	120	
Low fat, Plain	8 oz	100	
Low fat, Strawberry or Vanilla	8 oz	220	
Dannon			
Activia, Prune	4 oz	110	
Activia, Strawberry	4 oz	110	
Activia, Vanilla	4 oz	110	
DanActive, Blueberry, Cranberry/			
Raspberry, Strawberry, or Vanilla	3.3 oz	90	
DanActive, Plain	3.3 oz	90	

Protein (g)	Total Fat (g)	Sat. Fat (g)	Trans Fat (g)	Chol. (mg)	Sodium (mg)	Calcium (%)	Iron (%)	Carbs (g)	Fiber (g)
21	6	1	0	65	55	3	2	0	0
20	1	0	0	28	866	2	2	0	0
0	0	0	0	0	6	1	4	4	0
0	0	0	0	0	5	1	2	1	0
0	0	0	0	0	7	1	2	4	0
2	0	0	0	0	11	2	4	38	5
2	0	0	0	0	300	2	6	46	4
7	2	1.5	0	15	90	20	0	47	0
7	2	1.5	0	15	115	20	0	42	0
8	2.5	1.5	0	5	135	25	0	33	0
7	0	0	0	5	110	35	0	21	0
10	0	0	0	10	160	30	0	16	0
8	2.5	1.5	0	15	130	25	0	42	0
5	2	1	0	10	75	15	0	19	0
5	2	1	0	5	75	15	0	19	0
5	2	1.5	0	10	70	15	0	19	0
3	1.5	1	0	5	45	10	0	17	0
3	1.5	1.5	0	5	40	10	0	15	0

Yogurt FOOD NAME	Portion Size	Calories	
Fruit on Bottom, Apple Cinnamon	6 oz	150	
Fruit on Bottom, Cherry	6 oz	140	
Fruit on Bottom, Mixed Berry	6 oz	150	
Fruit on Bottom, Pineapple	6 oz	150	
Frusion, Cherry Berry Blend	10 oz	260	
Frusion, Pina Colada	10 oz	260	
Frusion, Strawberry Blend	10 oz	260	
La Crème, all flavors	4 oz	140	
Stonyfield			
Cultured O'Soy, Blueberry	6 oz	170	
Cultured O'Soy, Chocolate	6 oz	160	
Cultured O'Soy, Vanilla	6 oz	150	
Fat-free, Apricot Mango	6 oz	130	
Fat-free, Chocolate Underground	6 oz	170	
Fat-free, French Vanilla	8 oz	180	
Fat-free, Lotsa Lemon	6 oz	140	
Fat-free, Peach	6 oz	120	
Fat-free, Plain	8 oz	100	
Light, all flavors	6 oz	100	
Smoothies, regular, Banana Berry	10 oz	250	
Smoothies, regular, Peach	10 oz	250	
Smoothies, regular, Strawberry or Vanilla	10 oz	250	
Smoothies, light, Banana Berry	10 oz	130	
Smoothies, light, Peach	10 oz	130	

Protein (g)	Total Fat (g)	Sat. Fat (g)	Trans Fat (g)	Chol. (mg)	Sodium (mg)	Calcium (%)	Iron (%)	Carbs (g)	Fiber (g)
6	1.5	1	0	5	130	20	0	28	<1
6	1.5	1	0	5	280	20	0	26	0
6	1.5	1.5	0	5	120	20	0	27	<1
6	1.5	1	0	5	125	20	0	28	0
8	3.5	2	0	15	190	25	0	50	<1
8	3.5	2	0	15	135	25	0	50	0
7	3.5	2	0	15	125	25	0	50	0
5	5	3	0	15	65	15	0	19	0
7	2	0	0	0	35	15	6	33	4
7	3	0	0	0	30	10	6	28	4
7	2	0	0	0	40	15	8	26	4
6	0	0	0	0	100	30	0	20	2
6	0	0	0	0	100	30	0	37	3
9	0	0	0	0	140	35	0	36	3
7	0	0	0	0	115	35	0	28	2
6	0	0	0	0	120	30	0	25	2
10	0	0	0	0	150	40	0	18	3
6	0	0	0	0	105	25	0	28	3
10	3	2	0	10	150	40	0	47	4
10	3	2	0	10	150	40	0	49	4
10	3	2	0	10	150	40	0	47	4
9	0	0	0	5	170	25	0	41	3
9	0	0	0	0	85	25	2	41	3

FOOD NAME	Portion Size	Calories	
Smoothies, light, Strawberry	10 oz	130	
Yoplait			
Go-Gurt, Smoothies, all flavors	1 bottle	120	
Grande, all flavors	8 oz	220	
Grande, plain	8 oz	130	
Light, all flavors	6 oz	100	
Nouriche, all flavors	1 cont	260	
Original, most flavors	6 oz	170	
Original, Coconut Cream	6 oz	190	
Original, Pina Colada	6 oz	170	
Original, Plain	6 oz	100	
Smoothie, light, all flavors	8 oz	90	
Smoothie, all flavors	8 oz	190	
Thick & Creamy, all flavors	6 oz	190	
Whips! All Chocolate flavors	4 oz	160	
Whips! All other flavors	4 oz	140	
YOGURT—Frozen			
Ben & Jerry's			
Cherry Garcia, low fat	½ c	170	
Chocolate Fudge Brownie, low fat	½ c	190	
Half-baked, low fat	½ c	190	
Phish Food	½ c	220	
Häagen-Dazs			
Chocolate Fudge Brownie	½ c	200	
Coffee	½ c	200	

Protein (g)	Total Fat (g)	Sat. Fat (g)	Trans Fat (g)	Chol. (mg)	Sodium (mg)	Calcium (%)	Iron (%)	Carbs (g)	Fiber (g)
9	0	0	0	0	90	25	2	41	3
4	0.5	0	0	5	90	20	0	23	0
8	2.5	1.5	0	15	130	25	0	42	0
15	0	0	0	5	220	40	0	19	0
5	0	0	0	<5	85	20	0	19	0
10	0	0	0	10	270	30	15	55	5
5	1.5	1	0	10	80	20	0	33	0
5	3	2	0	10	85	20	0	34	0
5	2	1.5	0	10	95	20	0	33	0
11	0	0	0	5	170	30	0	14	0
6	0	0	0	5	120	20	0	16	0
6	2.5	1.5	0	10	150	20	0	38	0
7	3.5	2	0	15	100	30	0	32	0
5	4	2.5	0	10	105	10	0	26	0
5	2.5	2	0	10	75	15	0	25	0
4	3	2	0	20	65	20	2	32	<1
5	2.5	1.5	0	5	100	15	10	35	1
5	3	1.5	0	20	100	15	6	35	<1
5	4.5	3.5	0	15	95	15	10	41	1
9	2.5	1.5	0	35	140	20	6	35	2
8	4.5	2.5	0	65	50	20	0	31	0

Yogurt—Frozen – Zucchini, cooked, no salt FOOD NAME	Portion Size	Calories	
Strawberry, f-f	½ c	140	
Vanilla, low fat	½ c	200	
Vanilla Raspberry Swirl	½ c	170	
Stonyfield			
After Dark Chocolate, organic, nonfat	½ c	100	
Cookies 'n Cream, low fat	½ c	130	
Gotta Have Vanilla, organic, nonfat	½ c	100	
Javalanche, organic, nonfat	½ c	100	
Minty Chocolate Chip, low fat	½ c	140	
ZUCCHINI, cooked, no salt	1 c	29	
Raw, w/ skin	1 c	20	
Canned, w/ Tomato (Del Monte)	½ c	30	

Protein (g)	Total Fat (g)	Sat. Fat (g)	Trans Fat (g)	Chol. (mg)	Sodium (mg)	Calcium (%)	Iron (%)	Carbs (g)	Fiber (g)
5	0	0	0	<5	40	15	0	31	0
9	4.5	2.5	0	65	55	25	0	31	0
4	2.5	1.5	0	25	35	10	0	32	0
4	0	0	0	<5	60	15	0	20	0
4	1	0	0	<5	60	15	20	26	0
4	0	0	0	<5	70	15	0	21	0
4	0	0	0	<5	65	15	0	21	0
4	3	1.5	0	<5	55	15	0	24	0
1	0	0	0	0	5	2	4	7	3
2	0	0	0	0	12	2	2	4	1
1	0	0	0	0	490	0	4	7	1